PHYSICIAN, CARE FOR THYSELF

JESSICA WEI, M.D.

Physician, CARE FOR THYSELF

A DOCTOR'S JOURNEY Out of the DARKNESS of DEPRESSION and BURNOUT

NEW YORK

LONDON • NASHVILLE • MELBOURNE • VANCOUVER

Physician, Care for Thyself

A Doctor's Journey Out of the Darkness of Depression and Burnout

© 2021 Jessica, Wei, M.D.

Published in New York, New York, by Morgan James Publishing in partnership with Difference Press. Morgan James is a trademark of Morgan James, LLC.
www.MorganJamesPublishing.com

ISBN 9781631950179 paperback
ISBN 9781631950186 eBook
Library of Congress Control Number: 2020934008

Cover & Interior Design by:
Christopher Kirk
www.GFSstudio.com

Editor:
Nkechi Obi

Book Coaching:
The Author Incubator

Author Photo:
Jane Shauck Photography

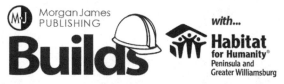

Morgan James is a proud partner of Habitat for Humanity Peninsula and Greater Williamsburg. Partners in building since 2006.

Get involved today! Visit
MorganJamesPublishing.com/giving-back

To all
Who serve tirelessly with their whole hearts.
Hold yourself with loving awareness always,
as you do for others.

Table of Contents

Preface

If you are holding this book in your hands right now, you may be experiencing symptoms of depression and burnout as a physician, or perhaps as a caregiver for others. Learning about another's experience is an excellent first step toward recovery and healing. To have some curiosity about the story of another who may share aspects of your own story can provide first glimpses into how you might find relief and freedom from how you are feeling now. I wrote this book from the perspective of a female physician and single mother who struggled with the challenges of practicing medicine while navigating significant difficulties with mood and energy. The ideas I write about in the book can be beneficial for anyone suffering from depression, anxiety, and burnout as one who cares for others. This includes most of us!

The premise of the book is that we all desire to live lives that are satisfying, meaningful, and happy. Yet, many of us find that no matter what we do, we cannot seem to find any lasting contentment. Instead, we may live from day-to-day from a place of constant worry about the future and what might happen if we don't try to influence the outcome somehow. With an inner and outer environment of constant pressure and demand, most find it challenging to relax into any sense of lasting peace in their lives.

This book was originally entitled, "Quit Your Job as a Doctor, Stat!: True Confessions of an OB/GYN Who Quit Her Job to Save Her Life." While this title does reflect some of the content of this book, it conveys some sense of an emergency. As if you need to decide at this very moment about your work life and your whole life. And there is no emergency, of course — my decision to leave my job as a doctor took many years of consideration. The sense of urgency conveyed by the original title refers more to the importance of considering what decisions you may need to make to save your life, to live a life you can truly love.

What I understand more deeply than ever is that the best decisions are made from our relaxed, centered, and grounded sense of self. When we continuously feel pressured and fearful, the choices we make are often reactive and impulsive. What unfolds in this book is the idea that to make wise decisions moving forward, we need to allow our bodies and minds to come back into balance and quiet. And yes, sometimes this movement toward calm involves leaving your job because that environment keeps you in a survival mode mindset, a near-constant fight-or-flight state of being. Unfortunately, this is especially true in the world of practicing medicine, especially in those specialties that keep doctors on the front lines of life and death decision-making.

I share the story of Dr. Jessie Wei so that you can understand that you are not alone in your experience, even if it feels at times that you are. Sharing our stories helps to loosen the grip of the false belief that we are ever alone. More than ever, we need to develop community and connection to support each other with love and kindness. For quite some time, I lived in the shadow of shame of the story I told myself about my experience that somehow I should have made different decisions. I now understand that I was doing the best I could with the tools of awareness that I had at the time.

And I am not my story, merely the one who experienced so much. Many of us suffer so much that we often or always feel overloaded with our fears and worries, and we forget who we are. We forget our capacity for joy and love as we feel buried beneath the weight of our thoughts and emotions. How do we start to remember who we truly are?

Begin with the idea you were not meant to live a life seemingly filled with sadness, exhaustion. Start to question any assumptions that you have about yourself and your life. Allow the words that you read to begin your own inner dialogue about what you need to shift into a life that you love. Make it a priority to cultivate the conditions in your life that continually lead to relaxation and calm. Know that there is a path out of the darkness of depression and burnout to the life that you are truly meant to lead, one filled with peace, love, and joy. There were hundreds of times when I felt that a life I could love was utterly out of reach. Little did I know at the time. The power to live my best life was inside me all of that time. And it is inside you too.

Jessica Wei, MD
West Hartford, Connecticut
January 2020

Foreword

I t is no secret that doctors are critically stressed and in crisis today. On the one hand, the technological advances of modern medicine have been significant, but they also have demanded that we physicians know even more than our predecessors. Add to this electronic documentation, insurance companies, and patients that are gathering information from many and varied sources on the internet, which often vilify doctors. Add to this the paradoxically longer work hours but shorter patient visit times, and this causes increasing layers and distance between doctor and patient. As hospitals and clinics become busier and more costly as the population grows sicker – this all becomes overwhelming madness. It is just not sustainable – even if doctors choose not to have families or a life outside of medicine.

I remember in medical school, all of the would-be doctors I knew went into medicine with a genuine, strong desire to heal. As doctors, we sacrifice significantly in the service of our calling – sacrificing our sleep, our youth, our relationships, our finances, and even, ironically, our health in the relentless pursuit to heal and deliver our best to our patients. But, unfortunately, we often find ourselves thrust into an overwhelming environment that makes it difficult to make the true healing difference we envisioned back in medical school. If you now have a family, you may be like me, willing initially to take on these sacrifices to "save lives" when you made that decision to become a doctor without fully considering the sacrifices that would be put upon your future children and relationships. It's not just us who sacrifice.

The negative consequences are high. The rate of physician suicide is more than twice the average for non-physicians! Yet, it is not uncommon for physicians to feel trapped – like they have no choice but to continue even if it is a dead-end. After all, what doctor in their right mind would quit medicine after all of the substantial investment of time, energy, and money. And what else is there? Could there be life after practicing medicine? Or perhaps we are numb to the consequences, having been immersed in a toxic environment where everyone else is doing it – so it must just be the way it is.

I remember leaving my twenty-five-year medical career as a radiologist at the top of my game professionally – even though I was the sole breadwinner for our family of six. As a doctor, I missed my four children terribly as I ran into the hospital on-call rather than tuck them in at night or watch them get awards at school. I was so deeply unhappy. But I saw absolutely no way out. I did not know of anyone who had left or how we would make it if I did. The costs of leaving medicine just seemed way too high – until that moment when I realized the costs of staying were even higher! I vividly remember that September morning, when I heard of not one but two of my colleagues who had committed suicide, and I immediately went in to see my next patient who was a doctor in whom I diagnosed with breast cancer! I'm next, I thought. I'm next! If I continue like this, this does not end well for anyone.

So, years ago, when I left medicine and "eventually" did find my way to create an absolutely fantastic soul-satisfying healing practice that gave me more time and energy (and money too as I followed my bliss), I had no support for this idea initially. I had no roadmap to follow. I felt like I was wholly disobedient and disloyal to my profession as I stayed loyal to my calling to heal truly. I desperately wanted "permission" to leave. I would have loved to have had a book like you are holding in your hands right now. I would have loved to know that I wasn't crazy or bad for considering leaving medicine. I would have liked some ideas or steps to take to sort out this big decision that I was facing.

I am so excited to write this foreword for *Physician, Care for Thyself,* in which Dr. Jessie Wei shares her story and perspective to which I believe all physicians can relate. Dr. Wei gives that permission that I was so desperately looking for years ago. She allows us to be open to the idea that we do have a choice and that our choices and our voices do matter. With love and kindness that is so characteristic of this amazing physician whom I have grown to know and call a friend, she shares with us that our health matters too. Doctors matter too.

In *Physician, Care for Thyself,* Dr. Wei will ask you to consider if you are on the path that you intended. She will outline some of the potential consequences of blindly continuing on your current path. She does not tell you whether to quit or stay with your current career, but rather to consider that you have a choice even though that choice may have previously been unthinkable. She also explores a unique fact about physicians – that our identity is so closely intertwined with being a "doctor." Often "doctor" is now included as part of our own name! Quitting your job as a doctor is a big decision, and it is so great to have a book like this to sit down with and assist you as you contemplate this major life decision.

One of the things I love best about this book is that the author dives into two factors that were essential for my freedom: the limiting beliefs that hold us back and embracing the uncertainty that allows us to move forward into something so much better than we could have imagined. I am living proof that this is possible. But as a "control freak" and as someone who loves "certainty," "safety," and "predictability" (like most doctors), that was initially one of the most challenging aspects for me. Outlining what that means and looks like as has been done in this book is tremendously helpful. Now years on the other side of my decision, this getting comfortable with uncertainty is not nearly as scary as I originally had thought. Now I love and welcome uncertainty as that is where all of the joy and fun in life live. I only wish that I had this book years ago to soothe and guide me through this important decision and phase of my life. Enjoy this book, my fellow physicians and caregivers, and I send my heartfelt love along with these words to soothe you during what is quite possibly the toughest phase and decision of your life.

But you – dear healer, caregiver, doctor – you matter, too. Your health and happiness matter, too. And you are not alone.

Be Good For You!

Shaunna Menard, MD
Author of *Free to Heal*
Founder of The Health Professional Academy 2019

Chapter 1:

Are You Sick and Tired of Working as a Doctor?

*"She awoke long before dawn and lay exhausted
and wakeful, with her eyes closed,
thinking of the countless years she still had to live."*
– Gabriel García Márquez, *Love in the Time of Cholera*

Sick and Tired

If you've picked up this book, then you're likely a burned-out physician like I was. Before I left my practice, I searched for and Googled all kinds of alternative jobs for doctors. I even considered working for a health insurance company reviewing claims – yes, I was that desperate to get out. How else could I use these skills that I had worked so hard to learn and earn? I just wanted to quit my job as a conventional doctor because I felt so exhausted and depressed. Yet, my deep fear about leaving my job and seeming stability prevented me from leaving for many years after I already knew I needed to go. And so, I continued to pay the high price of staying in a place that somehow felt safe and wasn't at all safe for me.

While your story is unique to you, I do know and understand the overwhelming and unrelenting stress of working as a conventional doctor while also attempting to balance the needs of family and home life. For a long time, I didn't think that I had any choice but to soldier on and live for the few moments of peace I had in the call room alone or my bedroom after putting the kids to bed. I felt trapped and miserable, and I became very emotionally sick with severe anxiety and depression. I also watched as colleagues became physically ill with seemingly innocuous symptoms such as digestive problems and serious illnesses such as stroke and cancer. It seems like the biggest paradox that doctors are becoming so sick while working so hard to take care of their patients. Yet, this is the reality that many choose and accept.

I Have Loved and Hated Being a Doctor

I have loved having the great privilege of listening to the stories of thousands of women throughout my career in medicine as an OB/GYN and functional medicine doctor. Because I'm a deep listener and a great observer of people and life, I've gleaned an immense amount of experience and wisdom about living life well and making difficult choices. I have had the great privilege of sharing many happy moments while delivering babies, meeting my patients every year for their annual exams, and celebrating personal victories, I have also shared the space of struggle, sorrow, and despair. In these moments, I have offered hugs, understanding, validation, and support. I have truly loved that part of my job.

I have also observed many other women while training to be a doctor in college, medical school, and residency, and then practicing as an attending physician. I have had many doctors as patients in both my conventional and functional medicine practices. Most of my colleagues were also mothers and wives and had a second full-time job at home. And of course, this was my own life as well as I've been a single mom for the past ten years to two beautiful sons. And one of the most common things we all often said was that we wouldn't have chosen this life again if we had the choice. Do we enjoy the privilege of being doctors? Often. Do we sometimes hate our jobs as doctors? Sometimes. Maybe, much of the time. We often feel that we don't have any option but to continue working at a job that demands so much of us. Yet, what if you do have a choice right now? An opportunity to live a different life, a life that you genuinely love.

Your Life as a Doctor and Caregiver

If you are a female physician juggling your job as a doctor and your responsibilities at home, then you are very likely feeling exhausted and overwhelmed, maybe depressed and anxious. You likely also struggle with physical symptoms and illnesses. And you may be wondering, short of running away and joining the circus (oh, I forgot your life already feels like a circus!), how do I possibly feel better if it seems as if I don't have the time or space to breathe?

Having children and being on maternity leave for six to eight weeks was almost enough incentive to have another kid just to have time off. Or perhaps the only time you've taken off is when you absolutely had to when you were so sick that you were forced to take time off. And vacation? It probably takes a day or two to be able to relax into being on vacation. Or maybe you can't take a full vacation because you have hundreds of electronic patient charts to complete. Or you're the one in charge of organizing everything on vacation, which means there isn't a moment to truly let your hair down and "relax." Or you don't take the vacation time you have because you feel as if you have to see as many patients as possible to pay your bills and support your family. Or maybe you are diagnosed with cancer. Even that doesn't slow you down very much. You may be so worried about letting your practice partners down and being away from your practice and patients for too long.

Maybe you were born into a family of doctors and professionals. As such, there was an expectation always to excel and perform. Training and becoming a doctor was the perfect means to prove that you were just as smart and capable as anyone else in your family. Or maybe you weren't born into a family of professionals, and there was the pressure to perform to rise out of the financial situation with which you grew up. Little did you know that medical training is expensive in so many more ways than just the cost of tuition. Residency training pays pennies for your slave labor, and private practice (especially as an OB/GYN) doesn't pay the bills as well as you need. The public perception is that doctors make lots of money, and that is more of the exception than the rule. The truth is that many doctors are struggling to pay off massive student loans (often hundreds of thousands of dollars of debt) while managing to pay a mortgage and other everyday financial obligations. Maybe you feel like if you made one million dollars a year, it might be worth the sacrifice of your time with your precious family and your sense of well-being. But even then, would it be? What is the actual worth of all that you've sacrificed and continue to sacrifice by being a doctor?

You Are Not Alone

In the 2018 Survey of America's Physicians published by The Physicians Foundation, a survey of 8,774 physicians revealed the following sobering and frankly disturbing findings:

- 80% of physicians are at full capacity or are overextended.
- 62% are pessimistic about the future of medicine.
- 55% describe their morale as somewhat or very negative.
- 78% sometimes, often, or always experience feelings of burnout.
- 23% of physician time is spent on non-clinical paperwork.
- 46% plan to change career paths.

What? Almost half of those surveyed are planning to change their career path? That's a lot of unhappy doctors trying to manage the ever-overflowing demands of work and home life to take care of patients. And we the physicians are the backbone of this health care system that often doesn't meet the needs of millions of patients. And the backbone is breaking.

The public conversations around health care in the United States mostly center around the issues of providing access to those who don't have access to healthcare and mandating that all Americans enroll in health insurance coverage of some kind. There are other conversations about how rapidly health care costs are rising or about how conventional medicine is merely sick care and doesn't meet the needs of chronically-ill patients. There are far fewer conversations about how sick doctors themselves are getting from practicing medicine. Why is this? It may be that we have the perception that if we as doctors reveal that we're having a hard time, we will lose the respect of our colleagues and our patients. Or maybe we're afraid we'll lose our license to practice. Perhaps we also believe that even if we did admit we're struggling, we wouldn't be recognized anyway to get the proper support we so desperately need. Moreover, our professional identity, or perhaps most of our entire identity is centered around being a healer, someone who holds power to help patients heal. If we admitted that we are struggling ourselves, what does that do to the whole dynamic of doctor and patient?

Yet, the truth is that doctors have been getting sicker and sicker as the days pass.

Doctors Are Killing Themselves

At the 2018 annual meeting of the American Psychiatric Association, the following findings were presented:

- Physician suicide rate: 28-40 per 100,000.
- General population suicide rate: 12.3 per 100,000, which then makes the rate of suicide among phy-

sicians as high as four times that of the general population.

- Female physicians attempt suicide less often than women in the general population, but when they do, they are 2.5-4 times more likely to kill themselves.
- Poisoning and hanging are among the most common means of physician suicide.
- Suicides are completed more successfully by physicians than by people in the general population because they have "greater knowledge of and easier access to lethal means."
- Of all medical specialties, psychiatry is near the top in terms of suicide rates.

Danger! Danger, Will Robinson! Danger! We are truly lost in space.

Have You Thought about Quitting Your Job as a Doctor?

It would be no surprise to anyone that you have thought about quitting your job and leaving medicine because it is a threat to your existence and life. Yet, you continue because you feel that you have no choice. Death or continuing to practice at a job that is killing you more quickly are not great choices. Moreover, there is a considerable cost for the decision you make to practice medicine. You already know this because this is your life every day. You hang on because you have such a strong sense of responsibility to your family and your patients. As such, your own needs get swallowed in a sea of confusion of so many competing demands on your time and energy.

A Story of Exhaustion and Illness

I recently started to work with a female physician who is in her early forties. Four miscarriages and then the diagnosis and aggressive treatment for breast cancer at thirty-eight have left her feeling broken and gasping for air. Yet, she continues to soldier on, working long hours at her practice, as well as taking care of her husband and children. She came to me primarily to address debilitating post-radiation fatigue, which isn't an uncommon problem during and after radiation therapy for breast cancer. It was so distressing to her that she couldn't recover her energy to live her life, and she could see that she was living in complete survival mode. What I found most striking were her answers to my questions about her "readiness to change." In functional medicine, we want to know that our patients are ready to make the changes they need to shift their health because if they're not prepared mentally and emotionally, lasting change will not happen.

While she desperately wants to shift back into having the energy to live her life on her terms, she doesn't feel that she has the space to change, even if for the better. She worries about taking time away from her husband and kids to focus on herself. She feels terrible every day of her life, and she believes that she is breaking down faster than she is meant to. She knows that it's from the "total life load" that she has put on herself, which is far too much. Ultimately, she thinks that "hibernation" is what it would take to get better. And she is right. Calgon, take me away! Calgon needs to take her away right now. How often have I wished that I had the magic Calgon bath powder to whisk all of us away to a secret tropical island to receive the care that we all truly need? Sadly, her story reflects the norm rather than the exception.

The Stories of Female Doctors

Her story is so similar to the story of many female physicians who feel entirely burned out and continually split off into the personas of doctor and mother to attend to the needs of others. They perceive that they have no other choice. And yet as the years pass, the body does keep the score. And what never comes to light is the bitter irony that doctors often do not have the opportunity or space to heal or take care of themselves. It doesn't come to light because telling the story of the shame of being sick while practicing as a doctor will reveal the crumbling foundation and could then threaten to bring the whole building crashing down. And we can't afford to have that happen.

So, we press on. And on and on and on like that silly Faberge shampoo commercial from the '70s.

For years, I felt trapped and powerless. I got sicker and sicker and sicker. I suffered in silence as I became more and more ashamed of how very ill I was becoming. Until I couldn't hide it anymore – until the building came crashing down around me. And to my utter disbelief and relief, this became the greatest gift of my life.

Chapter 2:

How Did I Make the Choice to Leave My Job and Feel Truly Good about It?

"Life is full of tough decisions, and nothing makes them easy...
Try, trust, try, and trust again, and eventually you'll feel your mind change its focus to a new level of understanding."
– Martha Beck

The End of Freedom at Age Five

I only remember one other time in my life when I publicly decided to "let myself go." When I was in kindergarten, I was the girl who carefully followed all of the teacher's instructions and always, always colored inside the lines. Until one day during playtime, the real class clown, Clara Joy, challenged me to push her around the large open classroom in the seat of a wooden baby stroller. I felt a bit reluctant, but she continued to egg me on, so I began to push her slowly around the room, maneuvering carefully around the other kids who were playing with blocks and other games on the floor. "Faster! Faster, Jessie! Push me around the room faster!" At first, I didn't listen until something broke loose within my good-girl self, and I began to run around the room, pushing the laughing Clara Joy faster and faster in the wooden stroller. "Faster! Into that tube over thereeeeee!" And without hesitation, feeling the thrill of freedom, laughter, and fun, I pushed her and the stroller into the entrance of this large, fluorescent, green, polka-dotted, flexible tube on the floor. Suddenly, there was the sound of children screaming, and my beloved kindergarten teacher yanking me away from the stroller. "Jessie! Go put your head down on the table over there! This is so unlike you!" Shame coursed through my body quickly like wildfire, making me feel that I had done something so unforgivably wrong, and I vowed never to break the rules again, not publicly anyway. And I put my freedom-loving, laughter-loving, and fun-loving self back into the box and locked it tightly shut. Never did I dare break the rules again. I continued to color inside the lines, and I started to look for ways to feel approval and acceptance always and at all costs.

Making the Decision to Go to Medical School

Growing up, I never thought much about becoming anything other than a doctor. My earliest memory of thinking about it was sitting in front of the television late at night. I would sneak downstairs around one in the morning and flip on the TV. I'd sit myself down on the brown and black shag carpet with the volume down very low to watch Sally Struthers, not in some reruns of *All in the Family*, but in some commercial program about helping poor children all over the world. There were so many children with sad eyes and bloated tummies. Night after night, I'd sit there with tears streaming down my cheeks, and this was a significant part of the birth of my wanting to help others.

My uncle practiced for over thirty years as an obstetrician/gynecologist, but I was sure I didn't want to do that because it seemed like he was always so busy at the hospital. He loved his job and his patients, and he loved his family deeply. I remember him fondly as smiling, laughing, and always being so kind to me. Very sadly, he died at sixty-four from a massive hemorrhagic stroke. His death was unexpected, and it was an unbelievably tragic loss for my aunt and my two cousins, and for his patients who loved him so much.

No, I was sure that I was going to become a pediatrician and take care of children. I couldn't seem to tolerate the sight of children suffering, and I believed that if I became a pediatrician, this would be the way I could help them. So, that was the thought that permeated my being and persisted throughout my school years as a kid.

You might think that it was my Taiwanese parents who pushed and pressured me to attend medical school, but it wasn't. When my mother observed the hectic life of her brother-in-law as an OB/GYN and its impact on her older sister's family life, she discouraged me from becoming a doctor. She gently said to me, "Jessie, that's a very stressful life, and I don't want you to struggle in that way." But because I didn't trust my mother or anyone else for that matter, I didn't listen.

I discovered along the way that I was the only one pressuring myself to do any of this. I had grown up in a stressful family environment where I didn't feel loved and accepted for who I was. I had been straddling the line as a first-generation Taiwanese- American being raised by parents who experienced an immense amount of difficulty and trauma growing up as children in Taiwan. While I now understand how deeply my parents love me, I didn't feel that way as a kid while experiencing significant and recurring emotional trauma. I had learned through some trial and error in my young life that performing well in school was a way to be recognized, acknowledged as smart and accomplished, and to be seen as worthy of love and attention. My parents did the best they could with the tools they had at the time, but I never really felt safe. I didn't know how to trust anyone, so I stayed in a survival mode state throughout my young life. My academic achievement was a matter of survival and acceptance in the world.

Attending Medical School and My Multiple Attempts to Escape

After my clinical rotation in pediatrics at the end of my third year in medical school, I decided that I didn't like the practice of pediatrics and dealing with the anxious parents of sick children. I unexpectedly fell in love with being in the operating room and decided that I wanted to be a surgeon. To my complete surprise, I found that I loved being in the operating room, and I loved being part of the surgical team. I felt a sense of belonging that I hadn't felt before, and I was hooked. I loved early morning coffee and rounds with the team, and I began to feel a level of acceptance and recognition I hadn't felt before. I specifically had my sights set on becoming a gynecologic oncologist, so I decided to pursue a residency in OB/GYN. Yes, this was the very specialty in which my mother and I had observed my uncle work so hard – the specialty I had said that I would never choose. I now understood why my uncle loved his job so much.

After I started medical school, any "subclinical" depression and anxiety had become very apparent. While I could switch on my excellent medical student persona on-demand to attend class and to study, I was much of the time almost catatonically depressed. From my third year of medical school, and afterward, I had been under the continued care of many psychiatrists and therapists for PTSD, depression, and anxiety. The primary psychiatrist treating me during this time had labeled me as having bipolar disorder and was unsuccessfully treating me with medication, even though I was pretty sure I didn't fit the criteria for this label. These were mere labels for how badly I was feeling. Nothing worked. Moreover, I had begun to have significant trouble sleeping, and nothing helped me to sleep, including hypnotics like Ambien, which helped at first and then stopped working. My body was on the highest alert, and I wasn't going to leave the watch or let my body rest or sleep.

My anxiety became more and more severe. I was in some kind of crazy whirlwind place, but I still was able to show up as a top medical student. I was twenty-eight years old, and I truly wanted to escape my life. I did everything I could to fail medical school during my final year, but I didn't. I accumulated three moving traffic violations during the two months I interviewed for residency, including a rollover accident during which I totaled my car. I felt and was nearly completely out of control, yet I was still able to pretend to be well and in control. I perfected this art of acting as if nothing was wrong when everything felt so wrong. I matched at the University of Connecticut for my OB/GYN residency and graduated from medical school with high honors. I somehow landed on my feet after spending the whole year trying to jump off this crazy train. And when I look back at pictures of my medical school graduation, I see that I have tears in my eyes and a look of marked distress. It was not a happy day when I graduated from medical school. I somehow already understood that I was on the path to disaster. Yet, the part of me that believed that this was the only way for me to survive would not let me get off this path.

I think you're starting to get the picture, right? I wasn't listening to myself yelling and screaming to stop, to get out of the way of the huge oncoming truck of being a physician. Does this story sound in any way familiar to you? The specifics are different, yet the overall themes of not listening to your feelings and inner being are likely very similar.

The Unrelenting Grind of Residency

I continued not to listen to myself during my residency in OB/GYN. If I was in survival mode during medical school, I'm not sure how to describe the experience of being suddenly thrown into the world of being called "Doctor Wei." I was learning how to be a doctor by working very long hours (up to 120 hours a week), with very little sleep, eating crap, feeling so much pressure to perform, and being criticized for not performing well. I was experiencing all of this while being entrusted to take care of the lives of other human beings. I often felt jealous of patients lying in their beds and simply wanted to crawl into bed too, lie down, and be a sick patient pretty much every single day. Yes, I was jealous of people who were ill enough to be hospitalized. You have had your own horrific experience of getting through your residency training. It's not pretty and is certainly something that is mostly hidden from the world. If I felt unseen before, now I felt completely invisible.

Love, Marriage, Divorce, and Checking Off Checklists

I married my best friend from college even though I knew that I wasn't in love. It was an apparent move to protect myself from ongoing arguing and conflict with my mother. He was my human shield, and I had always felt safe with him during college and felt threatened by the idea of being separated from him even though I was never romantically attracted to him. Since he was attending medical school at UVA, I chose to go to UVA for medical school as well. Finding safety at all costs was my priority. Nothing else mattered. You can probably predict that this first marriage story did not end well. We divorced in the middle of my final year in medical school after only five years of marriage.

Then, during my second year of residency, I met my second husband. And even though we were having trouble from two months into knowing each other, with repeated episodes of my crying and sobbing and feeling alone, I married him a year later because sometimes you can only do what you know. I got pregnant the next month, as planned, and gave birth to my first son by emergency C-section nine months later at the same hospital where I was the chief resident on Labor & Delivery.

I was hurling through my life faster and faster, checking off all of the boxes. Residency? Check. Marriage? Check. Have kids? Check. Finish residency? Check. Find a job? Check. Plan to have another kid eighteen months after the first? Check. I've been quite the expert at checking off boxes. This checking off of boxes felt good, at least.

So, I continued the life of checking off boxes. Build a successful private practice? Check. Have the neatest and most complete documentation in all my patient charting? Check. Be recognized as caring and smart? Check. Have David almost precisely eighteen months after Ben? Check. Be a caring and loving mother when at home to my two precious boys? Check. Oh no. Here comes something that was not on the checklist.

My mother became very sick in the months before David was born, and she was getting terrible medical care in Virginia, hundreds of miles away. I did what I could over the phone to help her while I was pregnant, on-call every few nights with a now bustling practice, with a toddler and then a newborn, and a very dissatisfied husband.

After I was finally able to help my mother a few months after David was born, I could eventually return to the safety of checking off the boxes. Study and pass my board-certification for Obstetrics and Gynecology. Check. Take fantastic care of patients. Check. Take overnight call in the hospital. Check. Take care of baby Ben and David when I get home. Check. Cook dinner. Check. Clean the house. Check. Bathe Ben and David, read to them, and get them to bed. Check. Take care of Jessie. Take care of Jessie? I was taking care of Jessie. I was. I swear. I was making sure all of the boxes were checked. That's how I believed I was taking care of Jessie. Check.

Fast forward to the winter of 2006. I was sitting alone again on the couch one night, over thirty pounds overweight, depressed, exhausted, overwhelmed, and I thought to myself: Is this the life you want, Jessie? Is this the life you chose? I realized that I had made every one of the choices that led up to this point of depression, exhaustion, no relationship with my husband, and a less than ideal one with my children. So, what different choices could I make? I decided to start with my physical body. It was the most natural and most concrete thing to focus on, and another thing to create checklists around. Perfect.

On January 1, 2007, I began an elimination diet after reading Dr. Mark Hyman's book *Ultrametabolism*. I joined a gym and started to work out regularly. I lost twenty-five pounds and began to have more energy and mental clarity. After I rode 1,500 miles on my bike during the summer of 2008 and completed my first century (100 mile) bike ride, I filed for my second divorce. I had already moved out of the bedroom and split our bank accounts at the beginning of the summer. After hundreds of miles on my road bike, mostly alone, I felt clear enough to decide to file for divorce. I knew that I wanted to protect myself and my children from the ongoing toxic conflict and irreconcilable differences with my husband. Then though, life became crazier and crazier as I felt more out of control with the dissolution of yet another marriage and breaking up of my precious family. But I was still able to show up reliably as Dr. Wei at this point.

Making Myself Sicker and Sicker While Practicing as an OB/GYN

In the spring of 2011, I had developed a large and persistent eight-centimeter cyst on my right ovary, not an uncommon finding for a stressed-out woman. After many months of waiting, I finally had surgery to remove it laparoscopically. The surgery went without a hitch; however, in the recovery room, I had excruciating pain at the five-millimeter incision site in my right lower abdomen, requiring a whopping twenty milligrams of IV morphine over the next hour for the pain to subside. My body was telling me that there was much danger ahead. My nervous system was on high alert, with good reason, because everything was about to break loose at work.

After taking care of myself and my sons during the week after my surgery, I returned to a full and challenging day in the operating room. I was placed on call three out of the next five nights in the hospital. During my weekend call, a woman arrived in labor. Although it began as a regular admission to the Labor and Delivery floor, it became a very challenging labor to manage. When the baby was very close to delivery, a placental abruption occurred, and the baby did not survive birth. The family was utterly devastated and in shock, as was I. The following week, one of my patients came onto the labor floor at forty weeks with the concern that she couldn't feel the baby moving. I immediately performed an ultrasound, which showed that the baby's heart was no longer beating. The baby had passed inside of her. There are no words to describe the experience of this moment. And I had the heavy burden of delivering this news as I had many times before to other expectant parents. I then delivered their beloved daughter with tears streaming down my face as I handed this perfect baby over to her to hold. There were so many tears and such deep sorrow. As if this wasn't enough, I also struggled with two more very complicated and challenging deliveries during the following two weeks. This is the work and life of an OB/GYN. I had never dealt with so many challenges and so much devastation on the Labor & Delivery floor in such a short time, and I certainly had never lost a baby during delivery.

To my great dismay and disappointment, I had little support from my practice partners at the time, who were also very stressed out and overworked. The only attention I drew from them was when I yelled at one of the nurses in the office. I had never yelled at anyone at work in the previous eight years. Ever. So, I was taken aside and taken out of the call schedule for six weeks and mandated to see yet another psychiatrist because I was told that I had PTSD that needed to be treated. This was the extent of the help I received, and all that seemed to be available at the time.

So much had happened. I had experienced during one month of my life more than any human being is supposed to experience in a lifetime. If I hadn't been broken open before, I was shot wide open now. During the emergency C-section for the baby I didn't save, I had begun to repeatedly mutter under my breath while I repaired the mother's uterus, "I can't do this anymore. I can't do this anymore. I can't do this anymore." Yet, I continued for another four years, taking obstetric calls, being on the front line of delivering babies and saving lives, and taking care of patients. And I continued to die inside more and more quickly.

Breaking Down and Breaking Open

Then, I woke up on October 1, 2011, and I proceeded to have a massive panic attack. I called out of work for the first time and was out of work entirely for the next month as I was ordered to go to an intensive outpatient therapy program to treat my "bipolar disorder."

In March 2012, I started to take a new medication that was a combination of fluoxetine and an antipsychotic in another attempt to treat the label of bipolar disorder. I slowly became less and less talkative, and I definitely didn't feel better. In fact, I started to actively contemplate killing myself and had stockpiled 360 tablets of Klonopin and multiple fills of different doses of Seroquel. I couldn't do it, though. The thing was I didn't want to leave Ben and David behind. I certainly didn't want to hurt them in any way. But I was determined to leave all of this pain behind, so I began to separate myself psychologically from them, telling myself that I wasn't a good mother anyway and that they would be better off without a useless mother like me. I had nearly fully convinced myself of that.

In late May 2012, I came home after being up all night with a woman in labor. A friend came over and noticed that I was "off." He was so concerned that he forced me to call the psychiatrist, and I was hospitalized because I finally admitted that I was thinking very seriously about killing myself.

My psychiatrist finally was in the position to dose me with lithium, the medication she had wanted to prescribe for years for the label of bipolar disorder which she had assigned to me. So that's what the inpatient psychiatrist promptly did. They stopped the fluoxetine/olanzapine, which had pushed me toward active suicidality. I was then very quickly dosed to 1,200 milligrams of lithium within nine days. On day seven of my hospitalization, I slumped over and passed out as I was at the window to take my medications. I had become severely hypotensive and was taken to the local hospital where the emergency department doctor quipped, "Don't let them give you so much medication." Funny and not funny at all.

I was discharged home two days later. I wanted to go right back to work because I didn't want to burden my partners with taking care of my patients and taking call for me. I didn't want them to be angry with me. But I wasn't allowed to go back to work for twelve weeks. When I met with my partners a few days after being discharged, one of them said to me, "You don't look any better." The anger and resentment from my partners were so apparent, and I again felt completely unseen. My needs were not important – definitely less important than their needs, so I believed.

During those twelve weeks, I attended another useless outpatient program, and I continued to have massive panic attacks despite being medicated with substantial doses of several medications. *The wrong questions were being asked, and the wrong answers were being given over and over again.* What I needed was to leave my medical practice to remove myself from the battlefield. Yet, I stayed because I didn't understand any other way to survive at the time. I also did not have any support to make different choices other than taking medication and returning to work.

The Final Straws: It Took Many Straws to Break My Back

When I returned to work after twelve weeks, I was placed on call ten out of the next twenty-one days. My partners were still feeling stressed, overwhelmed, and angry. I believed that I was a loser dud partner, so I did my best not to disappoint them any further. Meanwhile, I developed a tremor, and my handwriting became smaller and very shaky. Soon after that, my face broke out with severe inflammatory acne with huge purple and red bleeding nodules from my forehead and temple to my chin. My liver was shutting down from processing all of the medication, so I told the psychiatrist that I was coming off the lithium as quickly as I could against her advice. And within five weeks, I went from 1,200 milligrams to zero. I continued to be depressed and anxious, but my skin began to heal, and my hands stopped shaking.

A few months later, I came home from call after having to deliver by C-section, a woman who came into labor screaming for two hours fully dilated, refusing to push. I fell into bed exhausted and started to have vague pain in my left upper abdomen, which worsened over the next hour until I was screaming out in pain, just like my patient a few hours before. I was admitted and eventually diagnosed with a small bowel obstruction and stayed in the hospital for six days. An upper endoscopy revealed evidence of prolonged ischemia to my stomach from a functional bowel obstruction. This was likely due to the Seroquel that I had been taking for the past one and half years. I had been severely constipated for months. I had told the psychiatrist, but it wasn't considered a serious complaint.

Over the next two years, I got sicker and sicker to the point that I couldn't sleep at all anymore. I finally had to have the psychiatrist give me a medical order to stop taking overnight call because I was barely functioning at home while still forcing myself to perform at work.

I stopped taking call in December 2014. I almost took a job with a different practice, and then I decided that I was finished with being an OB/GYN. I gave my required nine months' notice to quit my job in September 2015 and finished working as a conventional OB/GYN May 31, 2016. I finally released myself from my self-imposed prison. And I certainly felt good about it. I was finally choosing to take care of myself differently than I ever had before. I gave myself the gift of space. I had finally removed my battered body and mind from the battlefield. This was when the journey to true healing began.

Why Share with You the Dark Shadows of My Story?

I just shared some of my story with you, as ugly as it is, to let you know that I know what it is like to believe that meeting the needs of others is more important than your own and to believe that you are taking care of yourself by pushing through everything that you don't want to do. I thought that I was keeping myself safe. I believed that if I kept checking off all of the boxes that I would meet my own approval and that of others, and then I would be happy. Yet, what I finally realized after hundreds of personal disasters, big and small, was that I was barely ever listening to myself at all. This is a repeated theme in my story. I would make myself well enough at times to keep going. We are so strong and so tough that we can continue to act against ourselves over and over again. And our bodies, minds, and spirits can take quite a beating. We take a licking again and again and keep on ticking.

Finding My Inner Clara Joy

As I started to study functional medicine in the fall of 2015 while planning to leave my conventional medical practice, I was learning about how our physical body and mind break down with chronic stress. I began to understand that I had been asking the wrong questions about how to feel better. If you're not asking the right questions, you can never find the correct answers. Studying functional medicine opened the door for me to look at how I was breaking down and dying more quickly as I pushed myself harder and harder. I had been in full-on survival mode since medical school and probably even since early childhood. I continued on that path of being in this chronic survival mind state until I learned how I was making myself feel worse and worse with all of the pressure to please, fix, and achieve. I finally learned what I needed to do to feel better and discovered a completely different way to practice medicine. I now had the tools that I had been looking for my entire life and medical career.

You are likely in a similar space right now, keeping your head just above the water while taking care of patients and your family. And you have no idea how to get out of this situation of being in continued survival and defense mode. When someone urges you to take the time and space to take care of yourself, you may not understand what they are saying. Even if you do understand, you don't know how because you have been very busy surviving your life, and you were never taught how to take care of yourself as a woman and a doctor.

Know that I see you and your struggles because I was there for many years until I woke up to my life. In writing this book, I have committed to traveling with you on the journey back to feeling good, with energy and mental clarity, so that you can live life on your terms. So that you can live the life you want to live, filled with freedom, laughter, and fun. Let's find your inner Clara Joy, who wants to laugh and play, to be truly free and happy. Start by knowing that it is possible. If, after all of the craziness of not listening to myself for so long, I can rediscover my inner joy, then it's certainly possible for you too.

Chapter 3:

How Do You Begin to Consider What to Do?

"Begin challenging your own assumptions.
Your assumptions are your windows on the
world. Scrub them off every once in a while,
Or the light won't come in."
– Alan Alda

N one of us intended to create a life of frustration, resentment, overwhelm, and exhaustion. You were not born saying to yourself, "Let me figure out how to live the most difficult and dissatisfying life possible and make myself sick in the process." And yet, this may be where you find yourself now after years of moving forward with training to become and being a doctor. So how do you begin to consider what you need? How do you find your way to the energy and clarity you need to make the best choices for yourself? Begin by scrubbing off some of your assumptions and beliefs, and you'll be surprised by the light that shines in.

The Path Ahead

In Chapter 4, we will begin to explore what questions to ask if you are considering or have ever considered leaving your job. Every process of discovery must start with the right questions. The main reason I never was able to recover from depression and anxiety was that I had not been asking the right questions to understand the roots of the problem. So, you will start by exploring the challenge of being a doctor by asking the right questions. Nothing to solve or answer initially. The first step is to be curious. You will be asked to use your discomfort, frustration, anger, and resentment to inform the questions you will ask yourself. In this chapter, we will take a look at the first two questions you can begin asking yourself. I will guide you through my process of considering these questions, and you will see that it is an ongoing process of increasing clarity and discovery. If you feel as if you don't have the energy or clarity to consider these questions, I understand entirely. We'll explore how to gain more considerable energy and mental clarity in the following two chapters.

In Chapter 5, I will review the basic physiology of the stress response, which we all learned in medical school, and then perhaps forgot about it. Understanding how we become trapped in the cycles of disordered and incoherent signaling within our bodies is the key to finding your way out of the darkness of living in survival mode and feeling much less than your very best. Conventional medicine pays some lip service to stress reduction and the role of stress in creating illness; however, the focus is still on treating the symptoms that arise from the disordered signaling within the body rather than creating coherent signaling. Letting your body know that you are safe is the critical and ongoing practice that will help to create the overall signaling and physiologic balance in your body that you need to feel better, have more energy and think more clearly.

In Chapter 6, you will learn about the functional medicine approach to addressing the root causes of the symptoms of exhaustion and overwhelm. Rather than working to categorize symptoms into a conventional organ system and disease diagnosis, functional medicine examines the underlying core imbalances in seven areas or "systems," each of which can contribute to an imbalance anywhere in the body. I will then take you through a step-by-step process to examine the "physiologic signature" of ongoing stress in your body, and what you can do to shift yourself back to feeling good again. You can do this on your own, but it's better to find a great functional medicine practitioner to help guide and take care of you.

In Chapter 7, you will explore why it's been so hard to choose to take care of yourself in the first place, and how it is that you allowed yourself to get to exhaustion and overwhelm. It's not as straightforward as telling yourself to love yourself and take care of yourself. To have any meaningful and lasting impact, you need to feel worthy of that love and attention. And feeling worthy and deserving of care can be a very complicated thing for those of us who don't fundamentally believe that we are worthy of love and care. We will review the first steps of remembering our worthiness and self-love. Without believing in your fundamental worthiness, you will return again and again to the same patterns of denying yourself the care you truly need, and then never discover the life you deserve.

In Chapter 8, we will dive more deeply into the question of why we resist taking care of ourselves, and why we resist understanding that our needs as just as important as those around us. We may laugh when people talk about "putting your oxygen mask on first." Ha! Right! At this point, you might be thinking that there is no way to focus on yourself first with all of the demands of being a doctor, wife, mother, cook, housekeeper, daughter, chauffeur, etc. However, when you pause for a moment to take a closer look, you see, and perhaps you already know, that your identity is so intimately intertwined with all of the roles you play. To let go of playing these roles, even just a little bit, seems so risky, so dangerous and unsafe. You hold on so tightly to these multiple personas that you don't even realize that you are living a life that doesn't feel good or make sense. You must put your oxygen mask on first and move out of the warzone of being in survival mode if you want to have any chance of feeling better. Chronically acting from a place of depletion will create illness for yourself and will impact the quality of care that you give to anyone else.

In Chapter 9, you will explore the limiting beliefs that may hold you back from deciding to quit your job as a conventional doctor if that's what you genuinely want to do. The truth is that all of us have developed all kinds of beliefs about what we think is possible and not possible in our lives. The noted psychologist and personal growth expert Gay Hendricks has described this as an "upper limit problem," a limited tolerance for feeling good. We will look at the possible limiting beliefs that may hold you back from taking the leap out of your current job. What limiting beliefs sometimes hold you back?

- I'm not good enough.
- This is what we do in my family, and I can't do it differently.

- Choosing differently will be more difficult than what I'm doing now.
- I don't want to seem like I'm better than others.
- I am afraid of failing.

We'll look at each of these more closely to uncover what might be holding you back from moving on from your job and living the best life that you truly deserve.

In Chapter 10, I will discuss the idea of becoming comfortable with uncertainty. Ultimately, for you to land comfortably with your decision to leave your job, you will need to learn to become comfortable with uncertainty. What? Isn't life about creating certainty to feel safe? Of course, we always have a certain degree of certainty and stability in our lives. And things are ever-changing. Not knowing exactly how things will unfold will be crucial to your ability to move forward with excitement and ease.

Finding Yourself and Your Freedom Again

Creating the ultimate sense of safety will allow you to shift into a space of true emotional freedom to choose what you want and need. When you make decisions from a place of a fully integrated sense of yourself, a place of unconditional love for yourself, you will be able to create the life you are meant to live. You need to take the first brave steps to see that this is possible. When you begin to see that the life you ought to be living is the life you are now living, you will develop the faith and confidence to move forward without needing to know exactly how it's going to turn out.

Ultimately, the story of your growth and movement will undoubtedly be very different than mine. I am stepping out of the shadows to tell my story because I want to let other doctors like you know that they are not alone. A big part of the problem for you may be that you don't feel seen or even believe that your needs matter to others. You may often feel like you don't have the energy or mental space to address your own needs. And this feels awful and hopeless. So, let's begin this journey by talking about what you might be facing and feeling right now.

Chapter 4

How Do You Leave Your Job When It's All You Know?

"Basically, the instruction is not to try to solve the problem but instead to use it as a question about how to let this very situation wake us up further rather than lull us into ignorance.
We can use a difficult situation to encourage ourselves to take a leap, to step out into that ambiguity."
– Pema Chödrön

The Massive Overwhelm of Being a Doctor

As doctors, we're trained to be problem-solvers. Patients come to us with their questions about their symptoms, and we try to neatly categorize those symptoms into a diagnosis and appropriate diagnostic code. Using that diagnosis, we then apply some algorithmic treatment plan, prescribe some medication, or maybe decide to perform a procedure. Sometimes the treatment works, and sometimes it doesn't. With this intermittent reinforcement of things sometimes working, we may continue in this way of performing our jobs because it works well enough. And then our jobs become somewhat mechanical and automatic with a set of answers we've learned. We may even feel irritated or bothered when patients question our answers and the solutions we've offered. This description is, of course, an overgeneralization. The point is that we're frequently focused on solving problems, and then often never look at the nature of the questions being asked.

I can only speak to this from my own experience of working as a conventional doctor. After years of traditional medical training, I had become an expert at gathering data from patients and making that data fit into a diagnostic category. Then, I would prescribe the remedy I had learned to treat that diagnosis. I always showed up intending to do my best every day and to listen as carefully as I could to what women were saying to me. I took as much time as it took to listen and to come up with a plan that made sense to me. Because patients don't perceive that they have much power in our medical system, they usually listen to what the doctor has to say and don't

question what is being offered. And we as doctors sometimes prefer not being questioned because questions
slow down our day, and it may even threaten our sense of
ourselves. Why is this patient asking me more questions?
Or who are you to question me? I don't have time for
this. The schedule of patients is like a checklist of things
to be done. Check. Check. Check. I've finished with that
patient. Good. Next?

During my years in the conventional medical world,
my job as a doctor became more and more pressured as
the years went by. The reality of medical practice is that
you need to see more and more patients to keep a practice running financially. It had been relatively simple to
keep up with the pace when we had paper charts and
forms to use to document quickly and move on.

Then, the introduction of the electronic health record
changed everything. You had to learn a completely different way of being a doctor. You had to learn a new
system of charting. You couldn't see as many patients
because charting electronically slowed you down so
much. You had to learn to navigate systems that were
not designed by clinicians, systems that made no sense
to doctors practicing medicine, and definitely made
practicing medicine much more of a burden. Those
requirements for documentation for billing became cod-
ified within a computer program, and the imposition of
"meaningful use" became yet another requirement and

checklist to grumble about and complete. And then, you became tied to the computer screen, concerned with getting the electronic documentation filled out correctly so that you could continue to move through and somehow get to the end of the day. That day often did not end until late at night or maybe on the weekend finishing the never-ending charting tasks. And during the time you were actually in the room with patients, you needed to look at the screen more than you looked at your patients. Patient care became even more mechanical than it already had been. Nothing you had any control over. Nothing you had any choice to do or not do.

If you were already feeling overwhelmed about practicing medicine, you became even more overwhelmed. The whole enterprise and intention of helping people became more and more of a burden. If you didn't have mental space to handle a person's questions about their diagnosis and treatment, you had even less mental bandwidth now. Because you have become so accustomed to pushing through and managing, you do that – push through. And there is a continued cost to yourself and to your patients. And often, you do not think that you have any choice but to stay in a system that does not meet the needs of doctors or patients. If we remain in survival mode, feeling trapped and having no choice but to continue doing what we're doing, patients often receive care that doesn't meet their needs. And, we are left practicing in an environment where our original intention to help has now been further diluted and confused.

Then You Get Home from Work, and...

Never mind what happens when you finally get home to your family, if you dare to have the dream of having a family. Exhausted and relieved to be home, at last, you start your second full-time job as wife and mother. The house is a mess unless you've allowed for the luxury of a housekeeper. The kids need to be hugged and loved and corralled and homework finished. Mail and email need to be checked. Bills need to be paid. Groceries need to be bought and put away. Dinner needs to be prepared and cooked. The dishes need to be washed. The floor needs to be swept and mopped. Mom needs to be called. The kids need to be bathed and put to bed. Your husband needs to be hugged and loved. Sex needs to be given...et cetera, et cetera, et cetera. Then, you fall into bed, and you sleep, or you don't sleep because your mind and nervous system are such high alert that you can't fall asleep or stay asleep. Then, the alarm goes off, and you start another day. Live for the little bit of time you may have with your partner, the weekend, or the time away on vacation when you can take a tiny break from your life as it is. It is during this short bit of time that you can breathe and have some relief from the machine that is your life.

And maybe some days, perhaps every day, you ask yourself, "Is this the life I wanted?" Or you may say to yourself that you don't like this life you've created. However, you feel like there is no other choice but to keep going because, after all, the bills need to be paid, and patients need to be seen.

Who Are You If You're Not Meeting the Needs of Others?

If you're anything like me, you are super strong and can push through most anything. Perhaps being able to push through becomes another badge of honor. Your life has become all about meeting the needs of others. The crazy thing is that you may feel that you need to meet the needs of others to maintain your sense of identity and worth, so to dismantle this machine, this structure, would mean dismantling your perception of who you are. And that feels pretty threatening when you are working so hard to keep it all together. Yet, the truth is that when your own needs are unmet, and you continue to ignore your own needs in the "service" of meeting the needs of others, you become angry, frustrated, resentful, and deeply sad. It's not possible to continue to ignore your own basic needs and feel happy and satisfied. It will make you sick.

So, what questions do you need to ask to be more clear about what you need and want? What is it you need and want in your life?

Start by Asking the Right Questions

The first step is to let go of resistance around daring to ask what you need and want. Many of us have created all kinds of defenses and denials to deal with the disappointments that started when we were very young. When you always prepare yourself for disappointment, for not getting what you want, you may eventually lose sight of what you truly want. You may have acted in the past based on what you thought you wanted only to discover that it wasn't what you wanted at all. And that's okay. Making mistakes is okay because it is the experience of trying that gives you more information about what you don't want. When you know what you don't want, you can understand much more clearly what you do want. Remember how I married twice, believing that getting married to these men was what I wanted when it wasn't what I wanted at all? I was so walled in by what I perceived I needed to survive that I wasn't actually in touch with how to get what I needed for myself.

There is no need or pressure to solve any problems right now. Allow your discomfort, frustration, anger, and resentment to inform what questions you need to ask yourself first. Ask the questions first without worrying about what the answers are. I understand that this is so counter to how we've been trained endlessly as clinicians. Yet, you don't need to have the answers right away. You simply need to ask yourself the right questions first.

> *"Genuine wisdom is knowing what we do not know; it is also seeing what is going wrong, although we may not always immediately see how to make it right."*
> – Dzogchen Ponlop Rinpoche

Start with These Two Questions

Two fundamental questions to start with are:

1. Am I doing what I originally intended in my work as a doctor?
2. Am I helping my patients in the ways I know that they need help?

I started with these two questions every day as I went to my job as an OB/GYN, and as I tried to make some sense of what I was doing in my medical practice. As the days wore on, I began to understand that I had unknowingly moved away from my original intention to help others, but not entirely, of course. The pressures of practicing medicine and meeting some seemingly meaningless and useless requirements of electronic documentation took me further and further away from my intention to stay present with my patients and to have the bandwidth and mental space to help them where they were.

As I observed what was happening, I thought that I could solve the problem by expanding my training, the breadth, and the depth of my knowledge base. Toward this end, I completed a fellowship in Integrative Medicine. I had a persistent feeling that I wasn't doing enough for my patients, that I didn't know enough to care for them as I well I wanted. After completing my fellowship, I did have more to offer to my patients; however, limited time with patients did not allow me to give as much as I wanted. In the end, this led to more disillusionment and dissatisfaction as I continued to see how I wasn't meeting the needs of my patients in a way that was lasting and meaningful. Moreover, I didn't want to be in the position anymore of being required to give the treatments that patients expected me to give as a conventional OB/GYN, such as prescribing oral contraceptives or unnecessary antibiotics.

I no longer wanted to practice medicine that required me to meet the expectations of easy answers to complex questions because it took me so far astray from what I had initially intended. I realized that I was unintentionally causing harm by providing the "easy" answers, and this realization ate away at me every day. I felt trapped and powerless even though I had been equipped with the best tools that conventional medicine could provide. It wasn't enough for me and it wasn't enough for my patients.

Because I thought I had no choice but to continue to practice in this way, I made myself sicker and sicker. I'm a person who stubbornly perseveres, and because I was very depressed and anxious, I had an even more difficult time extricating myself from my job. Considering leaving your job doesn't need to be that difficult or need to reach the extreme of having a severe emotional illness, cancer, or a heart attack. Even these events often don't move people to change what they are doing because it doesn't occur to them that their choices to push through are making them sick.

The answers to those questions may not yet be clear to you. To help you with this process, write the questions down on a piece of paper and write down whatever comes to mind, even thoughts like "This is stupid," or "I don't know." Write for five minutes without stopping. Simply start the process of looking at the questions. No problem is to be solved in this process. Start by being curious. If writing things down or journaling seems facile or useless to you, then simply close your eyes and reflect and daydream about the questions.

What Did I Discover after Exploring These Two Questions?

What I discovered in my process of asking these questions was that I could not help people in the ways that I had initially intended. What I noticed was that most women got a bit less or much less healthy every year. The most noticeable things I saw were that women were feeling more tired, gaining and not being able to lose weight, having more stressed relationships within their families, and becoming more anxious and depressed. Some would develop autoimmune disease or cancer. While I could offer a hug and some minutes of support and advice, I knew that there was not much more that I could do with the limited resources I had at the time. We had very little time with each other, and I didn't have all of the right tools anyway. Meanwhile, as I felt more and more out of alignment with my intention to help, I became more and more depressed.

At first, I was able to hold it together pretty well, and no one knew how I felt. Add to this sleepless nights on call and at home, running back and forth from emergencies, not being with or fully present with my dear children enough, fewer and fewer close friendships, and so many other stressors. I moved deeper and deeper into being in full-time survival mode. Finally, after getting very sick with severe depression and anxiety, I stopped taking the overnight call as an obstetrician. After fifteen years of sleepless nights, I began to practice solely as a gynecologist. I believed that this step back from the stressors of taking call would give me more room in my life to take care of myself. And it did temporarily give me more space in my life to breathe and move a bit out of survival mode. I was able to sleep in my own bed every night without being interrupted by phone calls and middle-of-the-night deliveries. I no longer had the responsibility of life and death in my hands, and this provided an immense sense of relief.

The thing is, though, once you wake up to something, you can never return to the way you saw or did things before. I began to wake up more and more to the fact that I didn't have the tools to care for my patients in ways that allowed them to feel better every year rather than worse. I also wasn't able to take care of myself in that same way. As I became more and more aware of the limitations of my conventional practice, I began to search for other solutions.

I Discovered That I Needed to Leave the Practice of Conventional Medicine

After starting my training in functional medicine in the fall of 2015 and completing yoga teacher training in 2016, I began to realize that I had to get out of the system of insurance-based care and leave behind conventional medical practice to create a new medical practice. In this new practice, I could incorporate all that I had learned to provide better and more powerful care for my patients. In many ways, my being an all-or-nothing kind of person served me well in that I didn't try to create some type of hybrid conventional/holistic care practice. My thinking was that there were thousands of gynecologists and far fewer providing the comprehensive care that I wanted to offer. So, I made the leap and left my private conventional medical practice. The truth is that when we distract ourselves with what we think we need to do while transitioning to a different type of work, it considerably slows down our ability to implement the changes we truly want to make in our lives.

Did Leaving My Job Make Any Sense? Absolutely

Did leaving my job make financial sense? To the world, it made no sense. I was a single mother with no other source of income. I now had an obligation to pay a sizeable malpractice tail, a lump sum paid to the malpractice insurance carrier to cover any future lawsuits that might be filed after I left my practice. My two sons were now in middle school. And I needed money to start my own business and functional medicine practice.

To be sure, the consideration of your financial situation is important. What is more important is living in alignment with your values and desires. What had become completely clear to me was that I was no longer serving my original intention to help others, and I wasn't helping my patients to be truly well. To live out of alignment, to walk beside yourself rather than with yourself, will not only create emotional suffering and unhappiness, it will create illness in your body, just as it does for every other person on this Earth. When you wake up to this truth, let it motivate you to start considering those two basic fundamental questions with more curiosity.

How Do You Begin?

You may not have any mental bandwidth to consider these two fundamental questions right now, and that's okay. You are where you are, and that is always good enough for this moment. For your well-being and health and that of your patients, come back to these questions when you can. At some point, you may understand that for you to meet your intention to care for others at your job, at home, and in every realm of your life, you may need to consider leaving your career as a conventional medical doctor.

It isn't easy to consider these questions, let alone consider leaving your job, especially the one to which you've devoted so much of your precious resources of time, energy, and money. It will be difficult to leave this job in which your very sense of identity is served by what you do.

As someone who made the leap, I will tell you that it was the right decision. To be free of the constraints of conventional practice and the confused and confusing system of insurance-based care has been frankly thera-peutic. After years and years of traditional care, drugs, and therapy for depression and anxiety, leaving the toxicity of my conventional medical job was one of the most significant gifts I have ever given to myself. It was this gift that allowed me to reconnect with my own needs and recover from my illness.

What gift will you choose to give yourself? Simply start with the questions first. It took me many years to reach the point of deciding to leave my job. What I also know is that I could have left sooner and saved myself many years of continued anger, frustration, and resentment. I also know that I didn't have the energy and mental clarity to make those choices at first. How did I get there? What can you do to address how you are feeling now? What steps can you take to improve your energy and mental clarity? Let's take some time to understand what makes us sick and tired and what we can do about it.

Chapter 5

Why Do You Sometimes Feel That You're Losing Your Mind? Because You Are!

"so much depends
upon
a red wheel
barrow
glazed with rain
water
beside the white
chickens"
– William Carlos Williams, *The Red Wheelbarrow*

What Makes Us Sick?

As you know, I was first conventionally trained as a medical doctor, then trained to be an OB/GYN, and became part of a private practice for thirteen years. During that time, I completed a fellowship in integrative medicine, and I am now also certified in functional medicine. I know firsthand how conventional medical doctors are trained, so I also know what I did not learn during medical school, residency, and private practice. My additional training allowed me to understand the underlying determinants of true health and wellness, and this is what I will share with you in this chapter.

While I could teach this in a very mind-based technical way, I am going to lead with my intention to create the conditions for healing in your mind, body, and spirit. When I was in medical school, we didn't focus too much on learning about the stress response even though all of us were experiencing massive amounts of stress. There is now more focus on managing stress in medical school education today, with the recognition that quieting and calming practices such as meditation and yoga help improve health and maintain a sense of wellness. But these are still applied like a Band-Aid over a gaping wound. It is not enough.

We must explore the roots of what makes us sick to understand how to feel better. *It is the ongoing imbal-*

ance and incoherent signaling within the body that makes us sick and keeps us sick. And the causes for imbalance are as multitudinous and varied as there are people on this planet.

The Basics of Survival

Your nervous system is taking in all kinds of information regularly from outside and inside your body to regulate your complicated and beautiful biochemistry and physiology. Threats of any kind are sensed in the brain by the amygdala, which then sends messages to the hypothalamus. The hypothalamus is the way station and command center from which inputs to your autonomic nervous system and endocrine system are received. The immediate response is to activate the sympathetic nervous system. This activation causes the adrenal medulla to produce epinephrine and norepinephrine to allow you to respond to a danger signal immediately. We all know this well as the fight-or-flight response. We also know what that feels like in our bodies, as either fear or anxiety. Soon after that initial surge of epinephrine, those sensory inputs are additionally translated into chemical signals in the hypothalamus. The hypothalamus then sends stimulatory hormonal signals to the pituitary gland, which then sends stimulatory signals to all of the other glands of the body. When there is a stressor sensed, the pituitary gland releases ACTH to the adrenal glands to signal the production of cortisol. This is what generally constitutes the hypothalamic-pituitary-adrenal (HPA) axis, the central axis of signaling, which governs whether we feel well or not.

You Are Completely Overloaded

Let's pause here to consider this. While we don't usually have conscious control over the automatic functions of our bodies, we do have the capacity to control how we respond to external sensory information. Therefore, we can control the hormonal signaling within our bodies. But we need to create the conditions to build this capacity over time.

The other point is that we are being bombarded with sensory information every second of the day, generating signals of stress and danger. There is so much going constantly, and your body isn't built to handle all of this constant information. And it wasn't built to withstand the chaotic experience of training to be and being a physician. What I am saying to you is that if you feel crazy, it's because your mind and body are operating in a massively imbalanced and incoherent state. And in that state, you cannot possibly feel well or think clearly on your behalf.

You can mostly operate automatically in your zone of competence while at your job because you are well-trained and habituated to performing your job well. Think though about when your patient asks you about something outside that zone of competence and habit. Do you ever feel irritated or uncomfortable or judge that patient to be difficult? Often this is because your survival-based self does not have any space to consider anything outside of what you habituated yourself to do. And this has consequences for the care that you can provide for your patients. I am not placing any blame here. I was there, and I see now how limited I was at times. I did the best I could with the tools and resources I had. I did an excellent job based on what I knew. I laugh now when I think about how I would react internally when patients would express to me their concern about having thyroid or hormonal issues. "Everyone thinks they have these issues! Stop bothering me! Your lab work will be normal, and I can't do anything about it anyway!" was what I would say to myself as I fake-smiled at the patient in front of me. I laugh because now I can see the irony. I now understand so well how we *all* have some degree of hormonal imbalance, whether thyroid or otherwise! I also now know that my living and operating from a survival-based stance in my life limited what I was able to offer to my patients very broadly speaking. While I practiced very well as a conventional doctor, what I had to offer was not what my patients needed to heal truly.

The Red Wheelbarrow You Can't Stop Pushing Around

Hormonal signaling throughout the body is much more complicated than what I've introduced here. Since we're talking about the mind and body being in a survival state, we'll focus on the production of the hormone we must produce to survive: cortisol. Cortisol is commonly referred to as the hormone of stress, but it is also the hormone of survival. Without it, we cannot live. Cortisol is the primary hormone in our bodies, which allows us to respond to acute and chronic stressors by releasing stored energy (primarily glucose) throughout the body, to give us fuel to act in a situation *perceived* to be threatening. After the adrenal medulla releases epinephrine and norepinephrine, cortisol is released by the adrenal cortex about thirty minutes after exposure to the perceived stressor. Pause here to consider that stressors must be perceived as stressful to be considered a stressor by your body. In other words, whether you feel something stressful is entirely dependent on your perception of that event. And perception is individual and ultimately modifiable through the practices of being quiet and curious.

When in balance, cortisol promotes the burning of body fat, maintains mood and emotional stability, counters inflammation, directs sex hormone production, and promotes healthy gut function. And unfortunately, if you are a practicing physician and a human being living in the modern world, you have disordered HPA axis function from the constant stress and overwhelm of medical practice.

It isn't merely a matter of whether you are making too little or too much cortisol. What matters more is that the signaling that your brain is communicating to the rest of your body is more often than not unbalanced and incoherent. Because you have so much redundancy and capacity within your body, you can handle the chronic stress for a while, and after a certain point of too much load, you will start to have symptoms. Sometimes this seems like a slow decline, or in the case of many who are in a chronically overly activated or overly sympathetic-dominant state, it will seem like your health suddenly changed overnight. This is because you've been pushing around a red wheelbarrow back and forth, in and around your life, loading and unloading all of the things you have to do and all the things you think you need to carry with you to feel safe. If you are so busy with focusing on the things that you are loading and unloading, you may not notice that your load is getting heavier and heavier, and the wheelbarrow that is your body is getting more and more worn down. You are so busy frantically pushing the wheelbarrow around and making sure your wheelbarrow is neatly organized and looks beautiful that you still don't notice that load is getting heavier and heavier. Then, one day, the front tire goes flat, and because you are strong and strong-willed, you still push that wheelbarrow around because your survival depends on it moving and carrying your stuff. You could stop to have someone repair the tire or maybe take some of the load for you, but you don't because your identity has now become so tightly tied to and associated with the wheelbarrow that you won't let anyone repair the tire or lessen your load. Then the tire falls off, and you get sick enough that you have to stop for a while. Maybe you are diagnosed with breast cancer or have a heart attack or stroke. And for a short time, you allow the tire to be put back on your wheelbarrow, and maybe the tire is even re-inflated for you. Once the wheelbarrow is put back together, you return to the same cycle of loading and unloading, running back and forth, because you don't know anything different than this. Consider this, though. You could decide to leave this overloaded and broken wheelbarrow life behind altogether because it isn't the life you're meant to lead.

What Does Overload Look Like?

So, what does a chronically overloaded wheelbarrow life manifest as?

- Less and less energy to do what you want to do
- Less and less energy to do what you don't want to do
- Digestive issues
- Food allergies and sensitivities

- Getting sick easily
- Gaining weight
- Losing weight
- Depression and sadness
- Anxiety and constant worry
- Insomnia
- Heavy and painful periods
- Hot flashes and night sweats
- Difficulty getting pregnant
- Decreased ability to remember and concentrate
- Irritability and being on the edge of overwhelm constantly
- And every single symptom you can think of…

The point is that all disease is the result of incoherent signaling within the body and that signaling begins with your perceptions and thoughts. If you are not aware of the subconscious habitual ways in which you are living your life, you can never change your life and truly heal. When you continue to think the same thoughts and support the same beliefs about yourself, you will never remember how to access your innate wellness, which you have within you all of the time.

So How Does Remembering Begin? How Does Waking Up Begin?

Because of the pace and "progress" of modern life, we are exposed to all manner of stimuli and sensory input that we were never meant to deal with: traffic, highways, smartphones, Facebook, Instagram, Twitter, grocery stores, fluorescent lights, computer screens, plastics, pesticides, electronic medical records, pharmaceuticals, malls, parking lots, EMF, talk shows, talk radio, news, newspapers, and being indoors and seated most of the time, and that's just what comes to mind in a few seconds. The volume of all of this sensory noise is enough to create hypervigilance, anxiety, and a chronically overactivated sympathetic nervous system. Then, add the content of what we're exposed to, and it's no wonder that many people are getting sicker and sicker. Once you add the cumulative load of medical training and practice to the energetic imprints of previous trauma and abuse, you've created the perfect conditions for burnout and illness.

Without really describing in detail how I experienced my childhood, suffice it to say that I developed into a hypervigilant human being who noticed everything in her environment. Any sense of safety was derived from being recognized as smart and helpful. I was very uncomfortable with external disorder, so I was a weird kid who cleaned up other kids' rooms when I went to get-togethers with family friends. It just made me feel better to put things back into the place where they belonged, and it felt good to be praised. That felt safe. I would straighten up anything that needed to be straightened up when I thought I needed a sense of order. Nothing wrong with that, right? Except that I was nearly wholly dependent on external conditions being perfect for me to feel safe. I was only listening to the messages I fed my brain and nervous system about what I believed to be reliable, what I needed to survive. Even when my body tried to tell me otherwise, I would ignore, ignore, and ignore. Shut up, body! Shut up, emotions! I'm trying to survive here. Just shut up! I now understand that this was profoundly confused messaging to myself. There was no way for me to heal if I continued to send myself messages to beat myself to a pulp regularly. It sounds crazy, right? And if you take a moment to be curious about your words to yourself, you might find the same to be true for you.

So, if disease begins with incoherent signaling which is triggered by sensory input and your perceptions, then the foundations of healing can be found by decreasing the volume on all of the high alert signals, and by increasing the parasympathetic relaxation signaling within your body. *You need to let your body know that you are safe and that your needs can be met.* You need to believe that you are safe. You need to learn how to create the conditions for feeling safe so that you can promote the coherent signaling that your body requires to function at its best. Then, when your body is working well, you will have considerably more energy and mental clarity, and you will no longer be living a life of reactivity to the endless cycles of crazy from chronically living in a state of survival.

Activating Relaxation Signals in Your Body

As you know, the majority of parasympathetic nervous system function is modulated by the vagus nerve. This is another aspect of health that has been largely underemphasized in healthcare. For a complete overview of the overarching importance of the vagus nerve and how to improve your overall health through improving vagal tone, please read *Activate Your Vagus Nerve* by Dr. Navaz Habib to learn how to bring more relaxation and healing to your body.

The vagus nerve, or the tenth cranial nerve, sends and receives messages from the lungs, heart, stomach, liver, gallbladder, pancreas, spleen, small and large intestine, and the kidneys. The outgoing messages to these essential viscera are parasympathetic and provide the brake and break from the sympathetic response. However, ongoing stressors and a negative perception of those stressors lead to less ability to activate that relaxation response in your body. As a result, the usual functions of your body are compromised, and you will experience increased inflammation, poor digestion (and therefore poor nutrition), less robust immune function, impaired detoxification, and increased rumination and worry, among many other issues.

Start to consider that your perception of what is stressful is modifiable through the practice of pausing, observing, and being curious about what is happening at the moment. The skills associated with modifying the lens of perception are best developed through the practices of being quiet and meditation, and through activating your parasympathetic nervous system.

How Does Practicing Conventional Medicine Lead to Further Incoherent Signalling and Confusion?

To succeed in medical school, residency, and practice, it is necessary to learn the pathology of the body and the associated ICD-10 diagnostic codes so that doctors can then understand what medications and procedures to prescribe and what procedural codes to submit so that they can bill for their services. Medical doctors accept this as how they exchange energy with their patients. In exchange for whatever codes the insurance company deems covered and billable, the doctor receives financial compensation for their time, services, and energy. The relationship between patient and doctor becomes a transaction in which what is being exchanged, and the value of what is being exchanged cannot be tracked. By contrast, in the days of fee-for-service, there was a transparent exchange of a certain amount of money for the services a doctor would provide.

Moreover, there was likely a strong relationship between the patient and doctor within a community in which people knew each other well. While some patients may still have strong relationships with their doctors, most care in the United States is provided through an insurance-based model with a less than transparent financial exchange between patient and doctor. Unless a doctor is paying attention, most don't know what they receive for their services, even if they happen to know what they charge.

Among other things, this confuses what is offered to our patients. Doctors are often not providing patients the best care by prescribing medications and proce-dures that usually do not truly address what is bothering them. They also are participating in a system where the energy exchange between human beings is convoluted and chaotic.

Why does this matter? It matters because this is one of the unspoken conditions which contributes to the "sick care" system. We live in a system where the expec-tation is that if you are provided health insurance by your employer, or you buy health insurance, then you will be entitled to some kind of care from your doctor. You don't know what the cost of your care is because all of it is pro-cessed through the insurance company. And your doctor doesn't often know what they are receiving from you for the care that they provide. When financial transactions are not direct, like when you go to Whole Foods and see that you can buy organic Lacinato kale for $1.99/pound, you don't understand the value of what you are getting and you might not place as much importance on what you are getting from your doctor. When doctors don't know what they charge for the care they are giving, they cannot understand the value or lack of value of the services they are providing. So, what exactly is being exchanged, and what is the value of that exchange?

I didn't think about this at all when I was practicing as a conventional doctor. I might have wondered from time to time what I received for a visit from a patient or for a procedure that I performed in the operating room, but most of the time, I didn't know. I had a large staff working with me to handle the vastly complicated world of insurance and medical reimbursement, so I didn't need to pay attention to any of that. When I left conventional medicine to start my cash-based, fee-for-service, functional medicine practice, I began to see and feel more acutely the disordered energy exchange that had been created by the expectation that medical care is paid for by health insurance. I understood how little people sometimes valued their health over other things when they had placed their health in a category taken care of by health insurance and conventional care. It seemed foreign to them that I might ask to be compensated directly for caring for them, especially caring for them in a way that would lead to the path of uncovering the underlying causes for their symptoms. While I understood how people had developed this expectation, I also saw how reluctant they were to invest in their wellness. They couldn't understand the value of the care that they were directly buying because their minds had not been trained in this way.

Likewise, when doctors participate in a system where they do not know what they are receiving for their services, they cannot understand the actual value of what they provide other than some vague sense of giving some kind of care. Attention is focused on getting through the busy schedule, charting, and surviving the day. I am certainly not saying that there are not many, many positive experiences that happen every day in the conventional medical world. I enjoyed many beautiful relationships with my patients and shared many smiles and hugs with them. But when I look back at what I provided for many of them, I realize how little I understood about a proper exchange of energy and value. If I knew what I know now, I would have been better able to provide the best care from a place of being my most integrated and happy self. Confusion begets more confusion. Lack of understanding leads to less and less wellness. We deceive ourselves if we believe that the way that care is delivered in this country makes any sense in most cases.

Calgon, Take Me Away!

It is no wonder that you are feeling burned out and overwhelmed, sick, and tired! You have been living and working in an environment of massively incoherent signaling and energy exchange. And this has taken an enormous toll on your body, mind, and spirit. It's time for a bit of Calgon shower powder, to take you away from this chaos back to a place where you can rediscover your energy and mental clarity, to a place where you have the power to take back your life.

Chapter 6

Physician, Heal Thyself? How Do You Begin to Heal Your Body and Mind?

"Love yourself first and everything
else falls into line.
You really have to love yourself
to get anything done in this world."
– Lucille Ball

Start by Cultivating Gentleness and Patience for Yourself

Waking up to your best life is a *process* with many ups and downs, twists and turns, and it takes as long as it takes. My wish for you is that you will be able to gather some of the tools you need to create the best physical conditions which will allow access to the best energy and mental clarity. I wish for you to have the courage to make the choices that you know are genuinely right for you. While healing ultimately resides within each of our minds and spirits, there are concrete steps to take to optimize the function of the brain and body to create the best conditions for healing. First, you start to turn down the volume on the signals of survival, and then you begin to create the conditions for coherent signaling in your body. Your body is crying out for help with the symptoms of exhaustion, weight gain, abdominal pain and bloating, constipation, loose stools, skin eruptions, anxiety, depression, irritability, crazy periods, etc. It's time to listen to those signals and learn how to pay attention to what they are telling you.

My best advice to you in this process is to find ways to be gentle and patient with yourself. Now, as I write those words, I am well aware that this is not simple advice to follow for many of us as we pressure and pound ourselves to accomplish all that we feel that we need to do. So, finding ways to be kind to yourself is also a process. We'll explore this more thoroughly later. For now, let's focus on some concrete steps for you to examine how being in survival mode has manifested in your body and then understand how to address those imbalances.

A Different Approach to Feeling Better: Functional Medicine

If you already are familiar with all of this, great! Read on to review and check-in with yourself. I am going to present the basic foundational approach to wellness that is the backbone of what we call functional medicine. What is functional medicine? More formally defined by the Institute for Functional Medicine, functional medicine is a "personalized, systems-oriented model that empowers patients and practitioners to achieve the highest expression of health by working in collaboration to address the underlying causes of disease."

Rather than working to categorize symptoms into a conventional organ system and then disease diagnosis, functional medicine examines the underlying core imbalances in seven areas or "systems," each of which can contribute to lack of balance anywhere in the body:

- Assimilation: what we take in and absorb into our bodies through our gut, lungs, and skin
- Defense and Repair: how we defend and restore our bodies, your immune system
- Energy: how we produce and manage the energy which we need for every process in our bodies
- Biotransformation and Elimination: how we handle toxins and eliminate them from our bodies through our liver, kidneys, skin, and gut

- Communication: how we manage to coordinate the massive amount of information the body requires to function through hormonal chemical signaling
- Transport: how we circulate information and energy around our bodies via our cardiovascular system
- Structural Integrity: how we maintain and repair the structure of our bodies to allow optimal function

Everything within your body works in concert with each other to maintain homeostasis and peace. Examining the function of the body in this way is a tool to look at things systematically and address the necessary foundations of wellness and optimal function of your body and mind.

You have all of the tools within you to feel better from the symptoms you have been facing. Once you uncover and understand the underlying causes of why you are feeling unwell, you can move forward to address those causes strategically. Functional medicine testing often reveals remarkable information that can unlock the keys to address health concerns previously challenging to understand. Having access to this knowledge is remarkably empowering and validating. Often people have been told that there is nothing wrong, and all of their lab work looks "normal," or they are given wastebasket labels/diagnoses like irritable bowel syndrome or bipolar disorder. Labeling or naming something does not then lead to the answers to why we aren't feeling well. It leads to the application of some remedy, which may address the symptoms in the short-term but does not examine the underlying causes for those symptoms. The harm with this approach is that the underlying process continues to progress, and its effects will manifest eventually with more symptoms and illness. This was my personal experience with the treatment of my emotional illness with conventional psychiatric approaches.

How Did I First Engage with Functional Medicine for My Healing?

My healing journey began back in December 2006 when I read *Ultrametabolism* by Dr. Mark Hyman, the ever-evolving functional medicine thought leader. At the time, I had just become a full partner with my OB/GYN practice, and my boys were two and three years old. I was working full-time, taking overnight call at the hospital two to three times a week. I lived in a large, beautiful house and had a shiny new dark blue BMW 330xi. I had it all, didn't I? Not at all. My marriage was breaking down quickly, I was the heaviest I had ever been, and I was more depressed than ever. Every night after completing my second full-time job as a mother, wife, cook, housekeeper, etc. I would plop myself down on the couch in the living room with a big bowl of Stonyfield Organic Whole Milk vanilla yogurt and mindlessly watch TV. I used to watch The *Apprentice* with Donald Trump and Omarosa. That's how sick I was! My husband would be locked away in his office, finishing up work, and I felt alone, depleted, fat, and miserable. I would ask myself, "Jessie, did you choose this life?" For quite some time, I simply felt trapped and unhappy and remained in massive survival mode because I just needed to keep my head above water.

One day, though, I realized that I had chosen this life and that I could make a different choice because we always have choices. We often convince ourselves that we don't. It is the fact that we don't like the perceived consequences of making difficult choices that prevent us from making choices that will lead to a much better life than the life we're living now.

I don't remember how I came upon *Ultrametabolism.* What I do remember is reading it and beginning to learn that I had the power to change my body and my mind. This was my first introduction to functional medicine, and it forever changed the course of my life.

On January 1, 2007, I took the first steps toward shifting my body out of physiologic survival mode. After I learned about functional lab testing, I had even more information and power to change my physiology and turn down the volume on survival mode in my body.

The steps I am going to lead you through are the steps that I direct all of my patients through to discover better balance and wellness in their bodies.

Step One: Pay Attention to What You Are Feeding Your Physical Body

The first step is to embark on an elimination diet. This is always the first concrete step because it's entirely within your power to start to turn down the signals of survival by removing those things in your diet that are creating the alarms, and replacing those foods with fuel that your gut and body can use to heal and thrive. One of the prime movers of an elimination diet is the reprogramming your gut microbiome, that second brain that lives inside your gut with the trillions of microorganisms that benefit you every day. By removing what hurts you and adding what supports you, you will be sending signals of safety to your body.

For at least three weeks (because this is the time needed to turn down the inflammatory/immune responses to the foods you are sensitive to), remove the following, which are the most inflammatory and allergenic foods: gluten, dairy (including eggs), soy, and peanuts. There are so many excellent resources to guide you on this journey, so I don't need to duplicate those here.

You will be surprised how much better you will feel simply by doing this. I've witnessed this repeatedly with myself and with my patients, and frankly, I'm still sometimes surprised by what people discover during this time. After just three to four weeks of implementing an elimination diet, women happily report better energy, better sleep, weight loss, less pain, improvement in digestive distress and bloating, better bowel movements, fewer skin rashes, improved mood, and periods, and much more. These were the very things I noticed after implementing an elimination diet back in January 2007. *So, yes! Just by changing how you eat, you can change the survival signaling within your body.*

To reintroduce foods after three weeks, follow these guidelines:

· Reintroduce only one new food at a time. Eat it two to three times in the same day, stop eating it, then wait forty-eight hours to see if you react in any way.

· Assess your response over that time, keeping track of your symptoms. If there is no reaction to a food, you can keep that food in your food plan and continue with the next food for reintroduction.

· If you are unsure whether you reacted, retest the same food in the same manner.

What I would say as a general guideline is that if you can generally avoid or eliminate those foods that are known to be pro-inflammatory for many people (e.g., gluten, dairy, eggs, soy, peanuts) then do that. If you decide that you want to know whether you can include certain favorite foods, try introducing those first. The other thing to consider is that food sensitivity is not a forever phenomenon. Once the gut and body are healed and back in balance, then often you can eat things that you haven't been able to eat for a long time.

Step Two: Explore Your Health and Life Story to Understand What Led to, Contributed, and Continues to Contribute to Your Not Feeling Well

When I trained with the Institute for Functional Medicine, one of the first tools we were taught to use with patients was a Timeline, a comprehensive review of their life story from birth to now. While I did take the time to gather a history with patients in my conventional practice, I had not been trained to review the timeline of a person's life from before birth to the present. This timeline provides critical clues to what led to the symptoms experienced now. It kind of seems like a "duh" to me now when I think about it. Everything in this life is cause and effect. While we cannot take into account every single event or cause in a person's life, we can look at significant events to understand what sets the stage for the manifestation of the symptoms of illness. When I meet with women for their initial consultation with me, we spend at least thirty to forty-five minutes reviewing their timeline story. What I can tell you after talking with hundreds of women is that *we all share the same primary reason for not feeling well. We are all living out of alignment with who we really are and want to be.* And when I see that fundamental issue it motivates me to continue to be curious about how to restore alignment and tune in to what really creates optimal health.

I am going to take you through what I do for my patients and why. I like to take a broad leverage approach meaning that I look for the processes that will have the most potent downstream effects on overall wellness, and this is what guides my approach. To find your functional medicine practitioner in your area, perform a search at www.ifm.org.

Step Three: Examine the Lab Data That Reveals the "Physiologic Signature" of Stress in Your Body

After listening carefully to a woman's story, I talk a bit of physiology with her, as in the last chapter. What I didn't discuss previously is that when the body is busy with prioritizing cortisol from receiving danger signals, the resource of pregnenolone, which is the mother hormone of all steroid hormones, can be siphoned away to make cortisol. This results in a decrease in the levels of progesterone, the anabolic steroid DHEA-S, and the downstream sex hormones testosterone and estrogen. When we feel as if we're running from a saber-toothed tiger, reproduction, digestion, detoxification, and immune defense are no longer priorities.

To understand the basic physiologic overview of what is going on with your body and the impact of being in chronic survival mode, you may want to explore the following lab testing with your functional medicine practitioner:

- Blood work:
    - fasting lipid, comprehensive metabolic panel, and insulin;
    - high sensitivity C-reactive protein;
    - complete thyroid panel including testing for antibodies to the thyroid;
    - complete blood count; iron studies including ferritin;
    - Vitamin D;
    - and a serum sex hormone panel around Day #19 of your menstrual cycle if you still have periods.
- DNA-based stool testing
    - This testing will reveal whether you have ongoing bacterial, fungal, viral, or parasitic infections that need to be treated to rebalance your gut microbiome, to decrease inflammation, and to turn down the danger signals within your own body.

- This testing also looks at digestive enzyme capacity, fat absorption, markers for dysbiosis, immune function through the measurement of fecal secretory IgA, reactivity to gluten (anti-gliadin IgA), occult blood, and an inflammatory marker called calprotectin.
- Comprehensive nutritional evaluation through urinary organic acid testing
  - Organic acids are metabolic intermediates that are produced in the pathways of central energy production, detoxification, neurotransmitter breakdown, and intestinal microbial activity. These can be measured in a single urine collection at the start of the day. Measuring organic acids allows us to understand whether your body is getting and using the nutrients needed for optimal health and function.
  - The testing that I use also measures plasma levels of essential fatty acids, markers of oxidative stress, antioxidants, and heavy metals.
- Dried urine hormone testing for comprehensive hormones
  - This testing looks at metabolized sex hormones levels and tells us whether the liver is processing estrogen favorably or unfavorably. 90% of estrogen-related cancers are

related to unbalanced metabolism and elimination of estrogen.

- Adrenal hormones, cortisol, and DHEA-S are also measured. The diurnal secretion pattern of cortisol can be examined to understand the ongoing impact of stressors.

Whether you decide to pursue this depth of testing is, of course, entirely up to you. The benefit of gathering this data is twofold:

1. Validation and explanation for you about why you have been feeling so bad.
2. Information that you can use as powerful leverage to find the vitality and energy you've lost along the way.

Is it necessary? No, it's not. However, because you are a physician in search of healing, this may be an essential step in your process of feeling better, finding more considerable energy, and mental clarity.

Step Four: Create a Comprehensive and Personalized Plan to Shift Yourself Back to Feeling Good Again

If you do decide to pursue lab testing, work with your functional medicine practitioner to leverage that data coupled with your personal story to create a comprehensive plan with supplementation personalized to your needs. The plan should focus on building a sound foundation for the healing of the whole body, mind, and spirit. Addressing stress is essential. Rebuilding gut barrier integrity and function is vital. The overall goal is to restore detoxification capacity, digestive competence, immune tolerance, and neurohormonal balance. When these basics are addressed, many other issues will improve or resolve.

The critical thing to remember and embrace is that we are what we eat, drink, think, and do. We all have the power to shift how we live and think so that we can feel our best and do our best in this life we have been given.

Addressing the needs of the physical body is just the first step to moving yourself out of survival mode. Once you are feeling more energy and clarity, this is the time to start examining what beliefs and mindset led you to create a life that you didn't want in the first place. Once you explore more deeply what has led you to make the choices you did, you can start to equip yourself with the tools and courage you need to make different choices to create the life of freedom and joy that you deserve.

Chapter 7:

Who Are You if You're Not Helping Others as a Doctor?

"I am not what happened to me,
I am what I choose to become."
– Carl G. Jung

How Am I Supposed to Love Myself?

You now have some tools to build an excellent physiologic foundation for feeling better. While it's a good starting point to have these tools, how do you move forward consistently in the direction you want to go?

Have you ever had the experience of starting with a good intention for yourself only to find yourself not following through? What is that about? Is it that you aren't disciplined enough or have enough willpower? This is very unlikely since you had the discipline and willpower to get yourself through medical school, residency, and now your medical practice. So, what is it?

What about this intention to "take care of yourself"? What does that even mean? Take care of yourself? Love yourself? Does it ever seem like the questions become empty or meaningless after a while because you have been told and have told yourself so many times to love yourself and take care of yourself?

I have had the experience of thinking that if I could just take care of myself or love myself, then I would feel better, and then I could be better. I've been pushing and pressuring myself to find the answer for how to do this, and I had plenty of other people telling me the same thing. "Jessie, just take care of yourself. Establish self-care practices. You simply need to love yourself." I heard it so many times and tried so many times to figure out this seeming conundrum that I began to feel angry when people would say these words to me. Why? Two reasons: it would continually reinforce the idea that there was something very wrong with me that needed to be fixed, and if it was true that I was broken and needed to be healed, I had no idea how to get there.

I had an internal and recurring story I told myself about all of this difficulty with self-love. I had a difficult childhood, like so many of us. While I've always intellectually understood that my parents loved me and took good care of me, I didn't feel the flow of unconditional love. I never felt like I belonged anywhere or to anyone. I was always waiting for the hugs and words of affirmation. Instead, I felt unseen, beaten down, and dismissed. How am I supposed to understand unconditional love if I didn't have the experience of it, and how am I supposed to flow love to myself? All that I know is that if I work hard and earn approval by being a good girl, getting good grades, following the rules, being neat, and being cooperative, then I'll at least feel like I am worthy of attention and love because I am behaving well and doing good things. I never questioned whether this was true or not.

I believed this to be accurate as I received attention for doing good things. I needed to do whatever it took to perpetuate the feeling of connection. I felt it most when I was in a romantic relationship, so that's what I'd do. I'd find the perfect romantic partner, and then I'd feel connected and happy. I'd think *I will create the perfect family, and then I'll be satisfied. I will earn and collect endless degrees and certifications, and then I'll be happy. I will be the perfect doctor, and then I'll be happy. Okay, I've done all that, and I'm still miserable, and I still feel unloved.* I could go on and on with the endless chatter in my brain. I felt so much pressure to continue to achieve and prove myself over and over again because nothing was ever good enough, and nothing seemed to fill the void within me.

You've probably experienced something like what I just described. The endless chatter and rumination is your effort to solve the problem of not feeling well. And because there doesn't seem to be a right answer, the cycles of suffering and feeling trapped continue. Why these ongoing cycles? Could it be that the solution does not lie outside the self?

Let's circle back to the idea of asking the right questions. I kept asking myself, how do I love myself when I don't know how to love myself? What is the question underneath the question?

Finding Hope

I couldn't understand the right questions to ask until I began working with a healer named Hope. The thing that seemed crazy was how I met Hope. I did not seek her out directly like I had multiple therapists, psychiatrists, acupuncturists, and other healers. I was simply following my bliss by taking a trip to mystical Sedona, Arizona, the first actual vacation I had taken in years. I met Hope after climbing a steep one-mile hike up to the peaks of Cathedral Rock. Both Hope and I live in New England, about one hour away from one another, so to have our first meeting between the magical formations of Cathedral

Rock was genuinely amazing. After finding ourselves in a part of the rocks that most people don't know about, we talked lightly only about how beautiful and breathtaking it was to be where we were. No personal details of life were exchanged. As I turned to hike back down, Hope looked me directly into my eyes and said, "I think you may need my help. You are facing some big decisions." Completely mystified, I blinked back at her and replied, "How did you know?" And thus started my journey with Hope.

Because I had opened myself up to find the real questions I needed to ask, I found Hope thousands of miles away from home, up high in one of the most mystical places on Earth. I had been asking with my heart, and I was ready to face the questions. The more important lesson to me here was that feeling good and finding bliss first led me to see and find what I needed. This was the opposite of what I had been doing all of my life. I thought that there were multiple checklists and checkboxes to complete before I could feel good. Who knew that I would find answers unexpectedly by feeling good and finding bliss first? And the more we step in the direction of feeling good, the more ease we have in our lives. This is simply the truth.

When I started to work with Hope, I was asking her questions about whether to close my current functional medicine practice. I could clearly and quickly see that I was repeating the same cycles of working, exhaustion, and depression that I had been experiencing in my work as a conventional doctor. This may or may not come as a surprise at this point because I ostensibly worked with root causes as a patient of functional medicine and a practitioner. What I soon discovered was that I hadn't yet addressed the real root cause of my exhaustion and depression.

Hope is an energy healer who uses her gifts of intuition to coach and uses energetic tools to uncover further the roots of feeling unwell. What we quickly discovered in our first session together was that I had developed the core belief at the age of six months that meeting the needs of others was more important than meeting my own needs. Not an earth-shattering discovery, right? And yet, it was critically vital to explore the roots of this core belief. The question underneath the question of how to love myself was: *what separated me from that sense of love in the first place?* What created this belief that meeting the needs of others was more important than meeting my own needs? The imprint of this mistaken belief led me to believe that all of the answers lay outside of myself.

Ask Why You Chose to Become a Doctor

Why did you choose to become a doctor in the first place? When you consider how difficult and challenging it is to train to be a doctor, you might wonder what it is that motivated you to become a doctor. A decision that forces you to continue to make choices against meeting your own needs over and over again. The basic requirements to sleep, eat, rest, and play are often ignored. For some, the decision to become a doctor may come from a truly grounded intention to serve others after feeling the love and caring from family and community. And for those of us who did not think or feel that we received this love and caring consistently, what is it that motivates us to act against ourselves and continue working against ourselves?

Exploring my core belief that meeting the needs of others was more important than meeting my own helped me to bridge the gap that I had felt all of my life between me and my sense of love for myself. I began to explore the idea that I needed to develop that core belief to survive during a time as a very young child when I needed to depend on others for survival. In other words, *I began to subsume my own needs to meet my own need to survive.* That doesn't sound like it makes sense, does it? It's confusing on its face. And then it's no wonder that I could never figure out how to love myself. I had developed a strategy early on to get my needs met by believing that by meeting other people's needs first, I would survive. Over time, the overdevelopment of this strategy to cope and survive led to the belief that my needs weren't as important, that I wasn't worthy of having needs. If this is confusing you right now, it's not surprising because the truth is that all parts of yourself *are trying to serve* you even though they seem like they aren't.

The Paradox of Subsuming Your Own Needs to Survive

Because we are very powerful and strong beings, we can act in such a way to completely crush ourselves with our thoughts and emotions, which then inevitably affects our physiology and our body's ability to take care of itself. We don't understand how to feel better because we don't understand that feeling unworthy and making the needs of others more important than our own is a very deeply embedded coping strategy. It is a strategy that doesn't serve us anymore and is very difficult to dismantle. It is impossible to dismantle if we never reach any awareness that this is what is happening. Without awareness of this convolution of beliefs, we continue to cycle through the same suffering and struggle again and again. And because it is a matter of survival, we pressure ourselves to find the answer and continue the actions and behaviors that intermittently provide some relief because it's all we know. This is the nature of habit and addiction. There is no judgment toward any being with any kind of addiction because this is often the only way we know how to cope with our pain and suffering – all of us, no matter how good things look on the surface. This was what I was doing in my life over and over again because I wasn't aware of what I know now.

At this point, you are either having an "aha!" moment, or you are very confused by what you just read. Both are valid experiences.

Cultivating Unworthiness to Survive

Let me repeat it: *I made myself feel inherently unworthy so that I could survive.* It doesn't seem to make any sense, does it? I developed the core belief that meeting the needs of others was more important than meeting my own to survive. I don't need to describe to you the conditions under which this arose because that isn't what truly matters. Assigning blame doesn't help because it places the locus of control outside of yourself as if you don't have the power to be well, or you need to rely on someone else or external circumstances to be well. The truth is that relying on external conditions – including the need to meet the needs of others to please others is a losing proposition overall, even though it makes us temporarily feel some relief. *The only source of love that can be reliably unconditional is your love for yourself.* Only you can flow unconditional love to yourself all of the time. Everyone is dealing with their issues of feeling separated and not enough. They cannot meet your needs unconditionally, and likewise, *you are not there to meet their needs unconditionally.*

Begin here: everything you do in your life is to serve your own needs. Through different experiences of distress that you did not know how to resolve when you were very young, you developed various strategies to deal with surviving that situation to maintain the connection with the people you needed to survive as a baby and child. Some of these strategies evolve into feeling self-hatred or unworthiness, things that don't look anything like things that serve your needs. *If everything you do in your life is to serve your own needs, you have a fundamental and intrinsic sense of worthiness to survive and to live.*

Reciting Positive Affirmations to Yourself Is Useless

Without getting to know and making friends with the coping strategies you uniquely developed to survive, you will not be able to uncover and remember your basic sense of worthiness that you were born with, a fundamental understanding of self-love. This is why positive affirmations alone do not work to shift your sense of yourself in any lasting way.

"Jesus loves me this, I know because the Bible tells me so." If you grew up in a Christian community, you might have learned this song in Sunday school, and perhaps in your own religious or cultural tradition, you have something similar to this song. It is a version of a positive affirmation, which is even more removed because now there is a religious book that is a stand-in for love! The point is that *simply telling yourself to love yourself or that you are worthy isn't enough to shift your underlying beliefs about yourself back to self-love and worthiness.*

Some First Steps Back to Self-Love

So, what are some steps that you can take to begin the process of uncovering your fundamental sense of worthiness and self-love?

Practice Pausing to Observe Yourself and Your Reactions

Be gentle with yourself as much as you can. Maybe you can't be gentle with yourself right now. I wasn't able to be gentle with myself for the longest time. That's okay because this is part of how you have learned to take care of yourself. Start by pausing to observe yourself and how you react to different situations, especially ones that feel difficult or disappointing. The purpose is to begin to bring some awareness to your thoughts and your emotions. If you think that it can be helpful, write these observations down. Noticing and having curiosity about yourself is the first step, even if it results in your being hard on yourself or judging yourself. If you find yourself thinking something critical or self-effacing, observe that. You can also say out loud, I'm judging myself.

Rather Than Resist Any Judgments or Self-Hate, Turn toward Those Feelings

Understand why the beliefs and feelings of unworthiness and shame are there and what they are communicating to you. Realize that while the beliefs are not true, they are valid in that they serve some kind of purpose. Admittedly, this step is best taken with someone who is experienced with guiding you through this process. You will want to find an experienced and profoundly intuitive healer who can lead and support you through this process.

Begin to Shine Some Light into Your Darkest Places

Begin to be willing to look at the places where you feel shame and guilt. At first, you may only be able to discover and share them with yourself. Eventually, though, when you dare to share these hidden beliefs and shame in a safe space, you will find that others are struggling with similar issues. Have the courage to tell your story. Be curious and observe in yourself and others how this need to survive and protect the many aspects of yourself can evolve into habits and behaviors that are no longer recognizable as the original need to take care of yourself.

Find a Safe Space to Share Your Feelings

Because I had developed a habit of not trusting anything or anyone, I didn't feel safe most of the time. So, how did I find a safe space? For me, it began with the decision to leave my job as a conventional doctor. My job was not a safe space for me to reveal my hidden coping strategies and my shame. I sought out spiritual support by attending meditation classes and spiritual retreats and eventually completing yoga teacher training. While I started to get closer to feeling safe, I still did not feel entirely safe because I still felt like I needed to hide. So, it was honestly a journey of trial and error, and gradually moving closer to finding a group of people with whom I could relate and who could see me. This is a realistic view of how this process unfolds. If there were a magic wand or secret potion to take to untie all the tightly tied knots of our confused coping mechanisms, then all of us would use these tools in a moment. However, what took time to develop and evolve takes time to recognize and untangle.

Set the Intention to Find Teachers and Mentors Who Will Help You

Ultimately, you will need to find teachers and mentors to help guide you because none of us know what we don't know or have no awareness of. We often need others to shine light and awareness on what is lying underneath the surface of the thoughts and behaviors that we cycle through again and again. We will discover that those behaviors and ideas that will never lead us to meet our deepest need for love and connection and, ultimately, to living a life that feels good and satisfying.

When you can be curious about what led to your choice to become a doctor, you will likely uncover that your most fundamental need to survive has become dependent on meeting the needs of others, taking care of others, and pleasing others. While you may have already understood this, you may not have realized that it is *turning toward the uncomfortable feelings of self-hatred and unworthiness that will lead you toward self-love and worthiness.* Begin to explore this idea for yourself, or at least plant the seed. By planting the seed, you will begin to tap into the growth and discovery process you will need to be free of the core beliefs that developed long ago. We can never know how long it will take to experience the full blooming of realization and awakening. It may take a few months or a few years. Know that the difficult work is worth the effort of finally being able to allow and receive the fullness of your self-love. When you act from a place of worthiness and self-love, you will have the freedom to make decisions that are indeed in alignment with what you need and want. You may just discover that you don't want to be someone who serves others as a conventional doctor.

Chapter 8:

Yeah, Yeah, Yeah. Put My Oxygen Mask on First, Right? Ha!

"You yourself, as much as anybody in the entire universe, deserve your love and affection."
– Buddha

You Don't Understand: I Can't Do That

Should the cabin lose pressure, oxygen masks will drop from the overhead area.

Please place the mask over your mouth and nose before assisting others."

We've heard it so many times while taking off on a flight that often we don't listen to the instructions from the flight attendant anymore. We put in our earbuds and zone out to our music or audiobook because we've heard it all before, and in our heads, we say, "Yeah, yeah, yeah. Right, my mask first. Right."

If you are a doctor and a mother, you might hear those instructions and say, "Whatever. That's not my reality." I have kids, a husband (or not), patients to see, a house to clean, meals to cook, soccer games to attend, parents to take care of, cupcakes to bake, obligatory sex to give, and on and on. I don't have time for me. Ever. So, while I understand the instructions, I know that I can't do that. I don't have any time or space for that. I have so many things to do and finish, and if I don't get those things done, then my life and the lives of others will come to a grinding halt, and that just can't happen. I'm holding it all together, and I have to take care of all of these other things first. That's the priority. Not me.

I get it. This was what I said for much of my life. I felt as if I was in survival mode all of the time with my head barely above water, the whole ship of my life barely above water. So it felt like life and death for me. If I don't get all of this done, people will not get what they need, and they might get hurt.

It begs and pleads so many questions, though. Why do we find it so challenging to take care of ourselves first? Why do we have so much resistance around the idea of making our needs just as important as the ones of those around us? What the heck is going on? And why am I so angry and resentful about all of this?

Survival Mode City

When I look at the world around us, I see that many people are living their lives from the mode of survival, meeting the basic needs of shelter, food, and clothing. In our world, making money and paying the bills becomes a matter of survival and continuing the life that we think we want to live. Being there for everyone in our lives is also part of our survival ethic because we believe that everything will fall apart if we don't show up to meet the needs of others. And then the more fundamental question arises, which most of us don't pause to consider: who am I if I'm not the one who meets the needs of others?

Who Am I If I Am Not the One Who Meets the Needs of Others?

One of the basic premises of writing this book is that people who choose to become doctors have their identity grounded in the need to be the one who meets the needs of others. It often is an attempt to solidify that identity so firmly and powerfully that no one will question it. Ever. If we anchor our identity with our training and profession, then no one can question our authority to say that we are ones who care for the needs of others.

And as we enter college and fulfill all of our pre-med prerequisites and watch as others fall away from that crowd, we feel good about ourselves. We have the academic prowess and perseverance to complete the classes we need and score well on the MCATs, accumulate all of the merits we need to apply and get into medical school. We become an excellent college student who overcomes all to get into medical school.

Then, we get into medical school, and we subsume our needs again in the service of the grind of getting through anatomy, anatomy lab, and the dissection of a formalin-preserved dead human body, biochemistry, pathology, pharmacology classes, etc. Then, we move on to the grind of our clinical rotations. There are so many hurdles, so many checkboxes, so many highlighters, so many pages of notes, so many sleepless nights, endless studying, and too many cups of coffee. And there may be so much resentment of the sacrifices made over and over. And yet, it makes us feel so accomplished. Even after seeing the faces of our classmates who didn't make it, we continue to press on. We steadfastly believe that this is the right thing to do for ourselves and for our goal of helping others. We become the persevering medical student who passes or even excels at the endless benchmarks of completing medical school. We must succeed at all costs because we may believe that our sense of identity and worthiness depend on our becoming a doctor.

We then match at a residency program and begin the long and arduous journey of living misery that is residency training. For those of us who trained before the institution of the 80-hour workweek back in summer 2003, many of us worked more than 120 hours a week, 75% of our lives spent at the hospital or clinic. When I completed my residency, I was paid $32,000 a year to work up to 120 hours a week — slave wages for slave labor. An education, yes, and absolute insanity. We get pushed far beyond the limits that any human being is supposed to endure, sleeping little, forced to do many things we don't want to do. We wake up in the middle of the night to the dreaded sound of a beeper summoning us to go to the emergency department or to rush to a patient "crumping" in the ICU. We systematically continue the mental training that is required for us to take care of patients. We become a soldier in the trenches, never knowing when the "enemy" will attack. We are merely part of the team, and we cannot fail to live up to the expectations of our team and our residency director. Failure is not acceptable, even if "failing" might allow us to save our own lives.

We then find a job as an attending physician and suddenly become responsible for the lives of others, as the captain of the ship. For those of us who were trained as surgeons, suddenly being the primary surgeon on call for emergencies becomes this real life or death job. We must show up to save a person's life, and suddenly we are the ones in charge. If a woman is bleeding out from a ruptured ectopic pregnancy on our first night on call, we have no choice but to move her to the operating room as soon as possible. We act as if we know with certainty that we can open her belly full of blood and save her life. We must develop yet another persona to handle every emergency and every problem we are presented with, whether in the office or the operating room. We feel as if we have no choice because who will save this person, and who will help this person if we don't? And we remain firmly entrenched in the world of survival. And it doesn't stop when we get home.

Does any of this sound familiar? This is one version of the life of a woman who has chosen to go to medical school, become a doctor, and dared to have a family. This is a story of living a moment to moment life of surviving, moving from one task to another with skill and agility. And we are part of the workforce entrusted to take care of patients. The fascinating thing is that we can do our jobs well in the face of exhaustion and unmet personal needs. Why? Because we have developed yet another persona to accomplish that, that of Doctor. We have learned to shift into yet another persona to serve the needs of others. And we do it so well that it continues to support the belief that we exist to serve the needs of others.

What Do You Mean the Splitting into Yet Another Persona?

I think we all instinctively understand that we have so many versions of ourselves that we have developed over time to deal with the many different aspects of our lives. On a macro-level, it may be that I am a daughter, a sister, a friend, a partner, a doctor, a surgeon, a mother, a cook, a housekeeper, a driver for my children, a sex partner, a runner, etc. Yet on the micro-level, it might look like something like this. I am a child who is seen and not heard. I am a child who is beaten and punished for no apparent reason, a child who feels profound shame. I am a child who becomes hypervigilant about the needs of others. I am a child with the need to please to avoid rejection and find a desperately needed connection. From these experiences are born multiple different personas to cope with all of these different experiences. And as we grow up and move into our adult world, we still carry with us these versions of ourselves which run in the background, in our subconscious mind habitually to the point that we're not even aware that these programs are running. You may be aware of this or not, and this is what is happening with every human being. The emotional and energetic imprints of our experience stay with us long after the original events occurred.

So, when we decide to become a doctor and solidify this identity as someone who helps others, we further solidify the ongoing belief that meeting the needs of others is more important than our needs. We believe that placing the oxygen mask on others first is more important than placing our oxygen mask. We believe that if we put our oxygen mask on first that we will die. What?

Read that paragraph again.

Examine the beliefs that give rise to the actions described above. What pushes you to do all of the things you do that you don't want to do? Most of the time, it comes down to your basic sense of survival. You believe that to survive – that is, not suffer – you must do all of these things that you force yourself to do. You are wired to value survival above all else. Stop to consider this, even just for one moment, if you never have. The first step in liberating yourself is to understand that you have come to believe that you don't have a choice to live this life differently because you believe deep inside that you will not survive if you don't live your life the way you live it now, as crazy as it feels.

The next step is to ask in the spirit of the teacher, Byron Katie: Is this true? It's not true that you will not survive if you don't live your life the way you have been living it. While you may say to me, "Of course I know

I'm not going to die!" trust that your body and mind function as if this is true. Otherwise, you would not be living the deeply unhappy life that you are living.

It is splitting off into the persona of Doctor (which has many other sub-personas) that has kept you trapped in the life you are living. And until you face that truth, you will continue in the cycles of suffering that you are experiencing. How do I know this? Because I did this for years until I discovered that I didn't need to do this anymore.

Why Is It Imperative that I Put My Oxygen Mask on First?

On the face of things, it seems like such an absurd question. Why take care of myself first? Why make myself a priority? Why consider my unmet needs before meeting those of others around me? The thought seems absurd. You don't believe any of it to be worthy of consideration because you are so hemmed in by all of the demands placed on you. I know I keep saying this, but it's a foundational thing to understand about yourself and every single human being on this planet, including all of your patients. Understanding this allows an understanding of what creates illness in your mind, body, and spirit.

It is imperative to put your oxygen mask on first because you cannot truly help others from a place of utter depletion. You believe that you can because this is what you've been doing your entire life, yet when you take a broader view, you will see that you genuinely cannot. The splintering of your persona to meet so many needs and demands is what has enabled you to do this for so long.

When you split off into hundreds of other personas to cope with all of the experiences in your life, you develop the capacity to act with the energy of more than one person, even when exhausted and burned out. Haven't you ever wondered about this? I have met hundreds of women who come broken down and depleted, and who continue to work and meet the needs of all the people in their lives. How do they do that? How did I do that? I could literally walk into my office, cry in the bathroom, wipe my tears away, put on my white coat, and see thirty to forty patients that day. How did I do that? Moving into the persona of Dr. Wei allowed me to do that, to tap into another reservoir of energy to be Dr. Wei.

The thing is, though, when you push yourself to live the multiple personas, and especially that of a doctor, you continue to deplete yourself of your vital energy, and your body and mind begin to suffer. Your body and mind begin to break down, and you further resist taking care of yourself as you fall deeper and deeper into the prison realm of living deeply in the world of survival first. As your body and mind begin to be out of balance, the signals of survival begin to grow louder and louder. Do you see that this a vicious feed-forward cycle?

You Know the Cost of Pushing Through Over and Over Again

The good news is that you aren't trapped living in this nightmare. It's just your perception that you are and that you have to stay there because if you leave, you believe you will suffer more. You can choose to move out of survival mode living into the growth and beauty of creation in your life. This is key.

You begin your life as a human being with this amazingly designed and complex physiology within your body to live and grow. Yet, as you get older, repeated experiences of stress and trauma wear your body and mind down until you start to have so many symptoms. You may be experiencing fatigue, heavy periods, digestive issues, getting sick all of the time, physical pain, hypertension, diabetes, heart disease, or cancer. Those symptoms are the result of the many years of the body coping with thousands of stressors. You feel awful, but you believe that you can still do your jobs and show up. You're amazingly strong like that, and much of your feelings of self-respect and worthiness are supported by your sense of yourself being ever able to push through everything.

Yet, this pushing through creates exhaustion, frustration, anger, and resentment. You force yourself to do things you don't want to do, and you force yourself to do many things that don't feel good in your body, over and over, day after day. After you continue to push through day after day, there may arise a sense of futility, meaninglessness, sadness, and depression. And yet you continue to say "yes" to things that are a "no" for you. This is the life that you chose when you chose to become a doctor. Not only from a sense that you wanted to be of service to others but also fundamentally from a feeling that your identity and worth are almost wholly dependent on being of service to others. The real tragedy, though, is not that you are doing this to yourself, it's that *you have not been aware of how you have been doing this to yourself.* And when you are not aware, you will not ever wake up to the life that you are meant to live – a life where you do things that you want to do, and you do the things that feel good. You might say that's not possible, as I did for many years, but I'm telling you, it is possible. If even one tiny part of you is interested in the possibility, then read on.

What Is Needed to Move Out of Survival Mode?

What you need to move out of survival mode is turn down the signals of survival and negativity. You need to move out of the environment of constant stress that signals that you are in danger. It sounds a bit exaggerated, but it's not. Your mind and body don't understand the difference between an actual immediate threat, like being in the direct path of an oncoming car, or an emotional threat, like the thought of seeing a patient who pushes your buttons and irritates you. The same stress signals are sent either way, and the ongoing damage is the same.

So, we can turn down the volume in two primary ways:

1. We can move away from the stressors; and
2. We can modify our reaction to those stressors.

Ultimately, I did this by quitting my job as an OB/ GYN. There was no way that I was ever going to heal by staying in the warzone that is Labor & Delivery, the operating room, the emergency department, and conventional medical office. This was the first essential and life-saving step for me.

What is needed first is to move away or reduce the stressors in your life. There is much focus on mindfulness practice and meditation as ways to address the ever-increasing stress in our lives. And while I agree that quiet practice and meditation are indispensable tools in the building and maintenance of a life you can fully embrace and love, it is impossible to have room to move if we are living in a literal warzone of constant incoming threats. We will fully explore this in the next chapter.

Begin to consider that when you choose yourself first and focus on healing yourself first, then you will be able to act and help others from a fully integrated sense of yourself. Until then, you can do a pretty good job of taking care of others; however, it can devolve to acting from a place of obligation instead of a place of true love. Over time, when you repeatedly operate from a place of "I have to do this" rather than "I want to do this" over and over again, day after day, you become exhausted, frustrated, angry, and resentful. Then your original intention to help becomes infiltrated with all kinds of other emotions that have the potential to create harm rather than good. You may begin to beat yourself up for the hurt you inadvertently cause when you are feeling overwhelmed with no room to think clearly and no space for yourself or anything else. Then, the inner anger and resentment come out when anyone suggests that you place your oxygen mask on first because you no longer even understand what that means. And when you don't know what that means, you have no access to the tools you need to heal and feel better.

And then you ask, how do I do that? Take the leap to leave my job as a physician? I'm glad you asked.

Chapter 9:

How to Take the Leap to Leave Your Job When You Don't Believe You Can

*"Always go with the choice that scares you
the most because that's the one that is
going to help you grow."*
– Caroline Myss

Who Likes Change?

One of the basic premises of this book is that nothing is rigidly locked in place. Nothing. While we can solidify our beliefs and think that we are not able to move out of those seemingly fixed states, we actually can. The first step is to pause to observe what we are experiencing right now. Pause. Slow down for a few moments for yourself. *If you do nothing else after reading this book other than to stop, to observe, and feel what you're feeling without judging or trying to change the feeling, that's a good start.* Even if you can only hold this state for a few seconds, it's a good start. What you will begin to notice is that you can do this for longer and longer periods, and that you find yourself stopping to pause to contemplate. When you open the door to your awareness of what is, there is no returning from that place. Eventually, you will know what you don't know, and you will be asking yourself the right questions to have your needs met. Now what?

The next step is to realize that you need space to move out of the survival mode life that you've grown so accustomed to living. You need to turn down the volume on all of the signals that keep you in survival mode signaling in your physical body and mind. This begins with the steps of attending to your physical body with the steps we outlined in earlier chapters. Start by pausing to tell your story, to be witnessed by another in your distress and overwhelm. Begin the process of knowing what has brought you to this point. Gathering the lab data that will reveal the physiologic impact of being in a chronically stressed survival state will empower you and your functional medicine practitioner to find the lifestyle and supplements you need to shift your body back into working for you rather than against you. Turning down the signals of inflammation and oxidative stress, and giving your body the necessary elements it needs to function optimally will allow you to consider what you need next. You may feel well enough that you will continue working at your current job, stay in your ongoing relationships, and continue to remain in the environment that has contributed to the noise of survival. And that is fine. It's your life with your choices to do what you want to do and what you think you're able to do.

This is what I did for years. I had addressed the physiologic imbalances through nutrition and lifestyle and felt well enough to stay in the same environment of my job and my marriage. However, because I didn't move away from those ongoing stressors, it was only a matter of time before the stopgap measures of attending to my physical body no longer were enough. So, first I got divorced, and that helped a great deal in turning down the volume. I continued as a single mother and full-time OB/GYN for many years, using romantic relationships to keep me afloat without considering that I was still in massive survival mode.

Eventually, the band-aid solutions that I applied to fix my overloaded wheelbarrow no longer worked. The wheel fell off, and I tried to push my broken wheelbarrow around with my will and brute strength. And my body started to revolt. For many, the seeming rebellion of the body manifests as getting physically sick frequently. For me, it manifested as emotional illness, depression, and suicidality. After years of trying to fix that with conventional medicine and then alternative modalities, I realized that I had not been asking the right questions about what I needed to do and, therefore, never found the answer to how to get my needs met in my life.

So much was related to having to handle the unrelenting demands and stressors of being a doctor. And while I had whispered to myself for years that I needed to leave, I could not conceive of how I would leave, how that was going to possibly happen. I daydreamed about being married to someone who could support me financially and emotionally as if that was the answer to getting my needs met. It seems like it, right? Thank goodness I wasn't in that situation because then I never would have woken up to what I needed to do for myself, or it would have taken much longer. *I began to see that not getting what I believed I wanted was actually a gift, the bridge I needed to have the life I deserve.* I became so uncomfortable that I had to examine what I really needed to change in my life. And it wasn't easy. No one is going to tell you that change is easy, especially when you decide to turn toward all of the things that have made you feel unsafe and uncomfortable in the past.

We all intrinsically resist change. We are all seeking safety and stability. And when we find a situation that is comfortable or comfortable enough, we will park ourselves there. To move into any other reality feels threatening because we are wired for safety and survival. We will move back instinctively to what feels safe, even if it isn't safe or beneficial to us in the long term. There is no blame or judgment about this way of being at all. We only know what we know.

What is also true is that if you never move outside your zone of perceived comfort, you will never have the opportunity to live the life that you are meant to live, the life you deserve to live. After working with many, many women in the functional medicine realm, I can see that we can attend to all of the physiologic imbalance we uncover, and women can feel great for a while to their great relief. What I've also observed is that for the women who hate their jobs and maybe even hate their partners and have other relationship stress, the symptoms and feeling unwell return very quickly. They feel better, but they have recurrent symptoms that seem to return no matter what they do. Could we dig more with more and more lab testing to find out whether there is some other physical reason for their symptoms? Sure, and what I know is that if we do that, we will still not be asking the right questions. And when you are not asking the right questions, you will never find the lasting solutions.

When You Say You Can't, It's That You Won't

In my practice, I often talk with my patients about the stress and pressure of their jobs and relationships. I hold the sacred space of seeing them in their distress and overwhelm. More often than not, my patients reveal to me "secrets" that they've never been able to tell anyone else in their lives. While all of them will acknowledge that this level of stress is contributing to their ongoing issues of not feeling well, almost all of them do not make the decision to turn down the volume of those ongoing stressors. They tell me that they can't. And while I understand their belief that they can't, I understand that this "I can't" is an "I won't." I won't threaten my current fragile state of survival and safety. There is an ongoing state of "grin and bear it" until it's financially safe to leave whatever situation they are in. There is deep fear that if they leave their job or toxic relationship that everything will fall apart, and then what? Again, it is a situation that we don't know what we don't know, so to stay with what we do know seems like the best choice, even though it is killing us faster.

No one demonstrated this more to me than my patient, Mary, who has taught fourth grade for over thirty years. After we began to work together to get her feeling better after developing severe colitis and then debilitating fatigue, she would intermittently feel much better, only to feel worse again. She was doing all of the right things: eating super-clean, exercising regularly, meditating, doing everything I suggested for her to do, but she still was having so many issues with digestion and sleep. While I advised her that she would likely continue to feel unwell while staying at her more and more demanding job, she didn't think that she could quit. Her husband had to stop working after having a massive heart attack. I understood that Mary wasn't quitting her job because the consequence of leaving her job seemed so much worse than if she stayed. Yet as one who quit her job, as a single mother of two boys, I can say that we don't know what will happen until we leap.

So how did I overcome the massive resistance to change, and make the leap? How can you do this in your life? It is a moment-to-moment process. When we establish and remember our intrinsic worthiness over and over and over again, we discover that we are capable of creating whatever we want in our lives. But how do we get to this understanding? And what's holding us back? Why do we choose not to live our best lives?

Taking the Leap

In his classic book *The Big Leap*, Gay Hendricks describes the problem of not choosing to live your best life as an "upper limit problem." An upper limit problem is the notion that you actually have a limited tolerance for feeling good. That sounds pretty odd, right? And think about it. Think about the life you've created to date. How much of the time do you find yourself in a state of feeling good? I'm going to guess, if you are living like I was, it isn't much of the time if you are a female physician with a family and children. Maybe 20% of the time? 10%? Only when you can finally sit down at night with a glass of red wine? What if I told you that we're designed to feel good most of the time? Could you believe that truth, and could you know that it's possible? This is another moment to stop to reflect about what it would feel like to feel good most of the time. What would that look like? Or do you even dare to think about that or imagine what that would feel like? Let's explore this further now.

You may have heard of this idea of limiting beliefs, those beliefs that hold us back from doing things that we want to do. We all have limiting beliefs of which we are aware. We also have those that we are not mindful of, running in the background of our thoughts and emotions, or in our "subconscious" mind. After experiencing disappointment or repeated disappointments from the moment we're born, we begin to believe that certain things are not possible. In this book, you are exploring the belief that it is not feasible for you to leave your job as a conventional physician even after deciding this is what you really want to do. Up to this point, we've looked at creating the conditions for you to consider whether you can leave your job by:

1. Shifting your body into coherent physiologic signaling; and
2. Beginning to feel your original and deserved worthiness to have your needs met.

Know that this is an ongoing life process that will continue to unfold. The next step is to look at your "upper limit problem."

We All Have Upper Limit Problems!

What limiting beliefs hold you back?

- I'm not good enough.
- This is what we do in my family, and I can't do it differently.
- Choosing differently will be more difficult than what I'm doing now.
- I am afraid of failing.
- It's easier for other people because…
  - They have more support.
  - They have more money.
  - They are smarter than I am.
  - They have more energy than I do.
  - They are braver than I am.
  - Fill in the blanks.

Looking at our limiting beliefs is not about creating another reason to beat ourselves up. It is about becoming more and more aware of our limiting beliefs and how to move past them. Like every other belief and habit you've developed in your life, it originated in service of you. So, what purpose do your limiting beliefs serve? Ultimately, you have a real need to feel safe. Let's look at each of the beliefs I listed above and how this has been a logical way to protect yourself. Remember, though, that the fact that something is valid doesn't mean that it is true. It merely explains why something exists at all as a belief or habit.

"I am not good enough."

This is the fundamental worthiness question that we addressed in the previous chapter. We explored why only having people tell you or your telling yourself that you are deserving and worthy isn't enough if there still exist other habits of mind always competing for airtime in your consciousness. We discussed examining these beliefs around worthiness to discover what information is contained in having those beliefs. By bringing those aspects back to yourself and releasing resistance, you create actual space for self-love and care to take root and grow.

"This is what we do in my family, and I can't do it differently."

This is a big one. Much of who you are has been determined by how you learned to cope with growing up with dysfunction. This is what we label *socialization*, learning how to fit in with the challenges you are presented with. You don't need to have any kind of extreme story of physical, emotional, or sexual abuse to have the ongoing experience of shaping yourself to the wants and needs of your parents. It could be as simple as being told, "Children are seen and not heard." Hearing this over and over again installs the idea that what you need to say isn't important and is enough to shut down your ability to speak up about what you need.

One of the most significant areas around which you may have limiting beliefs is your beliefs about money. Most of us were programmed with so many different and limiting beliefs around money. There is never enough; we need to work hard to save up for retirement; we can't do anything to threaten our ability to retire when we finally can rest and live our lives the way we want to, etc. These beliefs around money are the biggest obstacles to making choices to leave any job, even if keeping that job makes you feel downright miserable. The thing you don't stop to consider is the actual "cost" of staying in a situation that drains your vital energy. We believe that money is the only currency that counts in making decisions in our lives. This leads to the next limiting belief we'll explore.

"Choosing differently will be more difficult than what I'm doing now."

When we hold whatever limiting beliefs we have around money, we hold ourselves in a pattern. Because we perceive that making different decisions about our work will cause us to suffer in some way that is much *worse* than the way we are struggling now, we stay. It may sound something like this. If I leave my job, I won't be making money in a reliable way that I know that I am now. I may not make enough money to support myself and my family. I won't have the benefit of health insurance and a 401K to fall back on. I won't have enough. I'll lose my house, my car, and my life.

This all returns again to feeling safe. Yet, we often do not consider the other costs of staying in a job that drains us and doesn't allow us to meet our own needs. What about these costs? What were some of the things I realized that I was losing despite having a stable income and a job with the benefits we all believe that we need?

Losing time with my children as they grew up was a huge cost. I can remember countless nights lying in the call room at the hospital waiting to deliver babies, feeling sad, and separated from my toddler sons. When I was away from home for up to forty-eight hours at a time, I lost that time forever. And this was just the time spent in the hospital.

Even when I had precious time to spend with my children, I found myself having less and less bandwidth to handle the responsibilities of raising children. It was as if I had allotted a specific amount of energy to do the things I knew I had to do. If there were anything that arose that I didn't expect, I would feel ambushed and overwhelmed. What? I didn't plan for this! And I would sometimes channel the energy of overwhelm into yelling and complaining with my children. Only when I noticed the look of disappointment or sadness in my children's eyes was I then able to wake up to what I was doing. I found myself in this space over and over again until I found the courage to make different decisions. As much as growing up in my family made specific lasting imprints on me, I was creating different imprinting for my children. Ben and David are teenagers now, and I have had the opportunity to talk with them about not having this space, bringing awareness to how I know that this affects them. In this way, I have been able to address their wounding around my behavior. My yelling and screaming from a place of overwhelm was a cry for help, albeit entirely misplaced with my children. Thank goodness I woke up to this dynamic in my life.

Another cost was living a life that not many people could relate to. The truth is that no one truly understands what doctors suffer through during their training and practice. Living as my sensitive self and a person who didn't trust others to understand my needs, I kept my distance from developing deep and meaningful friendships. I didn't believe it was possible to have those kinds of deep connections because I felt so broken and like a literal alien whom no one could love. And the more I believed this, the more isolated I felt. While I never had issues meeting people to date and have romantic relationships with, I didn't have the energy or space to focus on the authentic foundations for a lasting relationship. I felt stuck in survival so much that meeting the needs of my partner and the relationship were priorities. I believed that my partner needed to meet me where I was. If he would only be the partner I wanted, then everything would be okay. I could not move out of this thinking for a very long time because, ultimately, this was about looking for that flow of unconditional love in places that I would never find it.

One of the other substantial costs to me was my emotional health and stability. I eventually knew that staying in the warzone of my work and personal life was never going to allow me to find freedom from my emotional distress. I had to leap into the void of the unknown to discover that leaving behind the insanity of my former life was the only way I was going to save my life. As I described earlier, I also knew that I was not providing the best care for my patients, perpetuating the cycle of suffering within our current sick care system. Ask yourself: *what non-money costs are you accepting in your life?*

"I don't want to fail."

Okay, this is a big one for human beings who have chosen to work as physicians. Failure is anathema to you and me. We've trained ourselves to achieve, accomplish, and surpass. How many exams and trials does a physician need to pass to become a doctor? Hundreds. On some level, while studying and training is challenging, these are very discrete and well-defined tasks to which we merely need to apply our discipline and knowledge to excel. However, to leap into the unknown of leaving your job is much more challenging. Without specific milestones to achieve, how do you measure success? How do you define success? Until now, success has likely been based on your ability to complete endless checklists to maintain survival in your life as it is. What if you were to consider defining success differently? What if facing uncertainty without the fear of failure was actually possible? We'll explore this more in the next chapter.

This is just the beginning of examining your limiting beliefs. It is a lifelong process of ongoing evaluation of where you are and where you want to go. Only when you feel comfortable with where you are, you may encounter roadblocks that don't seem to make any sense. It will be another time to step back to look at what limiting beliefs might be holding you back from living your best life.

Chapter 10:

How to Land Comfortably When You Take the Leap

*"And so, on this particular
Wednesday evening,
as Harold waited for the bus,
his watch suddenly stopped...
Thus, Harold's watch thrust him
into the immitigable path of fate.
Little did he know that this simple,
seemingly innocuous act
would result in his imminent death...
...And we must remember
that all these things,
the nuances, the anomalies,*

> *the subtleties,*
> *which we assume*
> *only accessorize our days*
> *are, in fact, here for a much larger*
> *and nobler cause:*
> *They are here to save our lives.*
> *I know the idea seems strange.*
> *But I also know that it*
> *just so happens to be true.*
> *And so it was:*
> *A wristwatch saved Harold Crick."*
> – From the 2006 film, *Stranger Than Fiction*

"Little did he know..."

When you have a chance, watch the movie *Stranger Than Fiction*. It's a story about a man named Harold Crick, an auditor for the IRS, who lives a very predictable and particular life of counting and numbers. And every day he lives is the same as the one before. Ostensibly, he is comfortable with his life as it is because he does nothing to change it. Until one day, he begins to hear an English voice beginning to narrate the details of his life while he is living it. While he is startled and disturbed by suddenly hearing this voice narrating his life, everything begins to change when he learns that his death is imminently near, apparently contingent on the fact that his watch has suddenly stopped. He becomes obsessed with understanding the source of this voice, which happens to be the voice of the writer character in the movie, Karen Eiffel, who has been writing a fictional book whose primary character is named Harold Crick. She has had writer's block for ten years and cannot seem to find the best ending to her book, how to kill off the main character, as she has in the previous books she has very successfully written. In the movie, of course, she doesn't realize this strange parallelism that as she is writing the book, the real-life Harold Crick is living the life she is writing and is desperately trying to figure out how not to die. And it is this uncertainty about when he is going to die that creates immense fear.

Yet, in his efforts to find out more about how he is going to die, he begins to live his life differently than he ever has before and stops doing what he's done in the past in an attempt to keep Karen Eiffel from writing forward any further. In the process, he begins to notice more about how he feels, in particular, that he likes and is attracted to a baker, Anna Pascal, whom he is assigned to audit. What unfolds in the story is the powerful idea that when Harold begins to act and think differently, *his life begins to open up in ways that he never imagined.* Although at first, he doesn't understand how to live his life more fully, he simply begins to take the first awkward steps. *He begins to wake up to the life he wants to be living, and thus his life is "saved."* He begins to live a fully engaged life full of love. He steps out of his illusory life of certainty to embrace full-on catastrophe, living that is so much more exciting and satisfying.

Little do we know. Or we don't know what we don't know. There is uncertainty inherent within everything because there is so much we don't know. For most, uncertainty about anything, especially about death, is very uncomfortable. Yet, the truth is that for you to move into a new way of being or even quitting a job that you no longer love or want, you will need to become comfortable with the uncertainty of what you don't know. That sounds pretty frightening, and maybe even impossible. How do you become comfortable with uncertainty?

Becoming Comfortable with Uncertainty

For me to decide to leave my job as a conventional doctor, I needed to become comfortable with the uncertainty of what was going to happen after I left. I was a novice in dealing with change at the time that I left my job in May 2016. Still, with more reflection, practice, and experience, I have grown to become more and more comfortable with making different leaps based on how I feel, as I tune into what I need and release resistance with myself. One of my favorite guides on this journey is Pema Chödrön, an American Tibetan Buddhist nun who is so incredibly skilled at using her own story of struggles in her life to guide others. She has written dozens of books, all of which I'd recommend you explore. One of the most useful on my journey has been her book, *Comfortable with Uncertainty: 108 Practices on Practicing Fearlessness and Compassion.* It is a starting guide on your journey to find the courage you need to leave behind your job as a conventional doctor, or anything that no longer serves you or brings you joy. Because like for Harold Crick, life cannot begin to open up until you face the discomfort of uncertainty.

My ongoing contemplation of being comfortable with uncertainty has been pivotally crucial for moving forward in my life with courage, faith, and joy. I now welcome change in my life.

Until a few years ago, I had been continuously seeking a sense of safety and security by having the unrelenting goal to make my life predictable and sure. I believed that safety was found in 100% predictability and certainty in my life. I thought that I could do this by checking off all of the boxes on my checklist of success. And so I did that. Yet I still hadn't been able to check off the biggest and most wanted item: to feel happy and satisfied with my life. I seemed to have failed miserably at being happy and satisfied.

What happened? I had been able to check off all of the boxes relatively quickly. I didn't treat myself well during that time, but what did that have to do with anything? All that mattered was getting through my perfect checklist. Even though I was becoming more and more depressed as the years passed, I still was able to push myself through all of it because I believed that my life would be so much worse if I didn't push through. I honestly thought that it was a matter of survival. I look back at that time now, and it astounds me. I have also now witnessed this very same dynamic with so many women in my functional medicine practice, especially with female physicians and other women working in the professional world. I truly believed with all of my being that if I moved heaven and earth to accomplish everything on the checklist that there would be a chocolate ice cream sundae with whipped cream and a bright red maraschino cherry on top waiting for me at the end of the rainbow with unicorns and butterflies everywhere... And all would be well. In other words, it was a dream and, ultimately, an illusory fairytale. I believed and told myself over and over again to push ahead. I thought that comfort was created from the perceived security of certainty. Yet, the more I drove in this direction, the more dissatisfied and depressed I became.

The Truth Is That Certainty Is Never Attainable

The only thing that is ever certain is that nothing is truly solid or lasting, and we can never know what the next moment will hold. This not knowing is what can create an immense sense of fear and dread for many of us. Will I be mugged when I ride the subway in the city? Will the stock market crash and obliterate my 401K? Will they run out of my favorite kale chips at Whole Foods? Will five women come into labor when I'm on call tonight? Will my boss destroy me if I don't meet my deadline? Will my husband ever love and touch me in the way that I want? It sounds a bit absurd, and yet, stop to notice your thoughts and how people generally talk about their lives. There is so much fear about the future. As such, there is also constant striving to maintain the structure of life as it is now, to attempt to keep a sense of safety and certainty. When you pause to consider this, it becomes evident that this is an incredibly fragile and precariously dangerous way to live. And you might say that you're "realistic," and I would say that's not real or realistic at all. Any reality that hinges on external conditions to be "just right" is a very unsafe way to live because it relies on the delusion that we can ever be in complete control of anything outside of ourselves. And then, as such, we are destined to fail. A happy and satisfying life never appears to be within reach.

How Do You Become Comfortable with Uncertainty?

If you want to loosen the ties you have with wanting certainty as much as I had wanted it in the past, start with observing when something surprising happens in your life. It's easiest to start with unexpected things that you make you feel happy. A close friend calls you out of the blue. Your partner buys you a beautiful bouquet for no particular reason. Your favorite kale chips are on sale at Whole Foods. You are given a raise at work that you weren't expecting. There were surprises, so there wasn't any certainty in those things happening during your day, and they made you feel lucky and happy. You welcome this kind of uncertainty in your life. Because it feels enjoyable and exciting, feeling comfortable with this kind of uncertainty is pretty straightforward. I love recognizing this and having immense gratitude when unexpected gifts come my way. It happens every day and happens more, and more consistently, the more I open myself up to the appreciation I have for these moments.

How about when something upsetting happens unexpectedly? Your mother is diagnosed with a severe and debilitating bone infection, just as your second son is born. You have a screaming and yelling argument with your husband after spending all day preparing his favorite meal. Your car is rear-ended amidst crazy traffic as you are driving home from a long day at work. It is admittedly far more challenging to see the gifts in these situations. What gifts? These are terrible things, aren't they? They certainly don't feel good at the time they happen. Yet, this is life unfolding as well. And as my awareness began to expand, I began to appreciate that when seemingly "negative" things happened in my life, there was a gift within each of these things, some profound wisdom and deeper awareness that came with these events if I could pause to reflect.

My mother came through that harrowing time in her life when she had debilitating pain from that bone infection with more in-depth knowledge about how to take the best care of herself. If you ask her today, she will tell you that she is much healthier than before her time of serious illness, and she feels so much better than before all of that happened to her body. And had that never happened, she likely would not be in the excellent health she is in now. That argument with your husband? It is either helpful information for you or an opportunity for both of you to reconnect because negative emotion tells you very clearly what you don't want. The car accident gives you a chance to observe your reactions, skillful or unskillful, and whether you increased your suffering and that of the other driver. Facing the thought of imminent death, as Harold Crick did in the movie, creates the space for all manner of realization and commitment to living what you want to live.

Consider the Freedom of Choice

If you have the openness and courage to work and practice with this view of all things happening as opportunities, you will develop the power to live a life with authentic emotional freedom. For most of my life, I saw myself as a victim of circumstance, powerless against the seeming unfairness of life. It was only when I began to open myself up to noticing my feelings and thoughts that the window of greater awareness opened. I realized that I was making choices that led to that current reality of my life, and I had the power to make different choices. I began to let everything be my teacher, whatever appeared, "good" or "bad." In the end, there is no good or bad. It's all helpful information on your path.

I began to discover that feeling good and having my needs met wasn't about doing anything or mentally checking off boxes on a list of what I thought I needed to do. It became a process of feeling good first, then watching what arose from that place of feeling good. I realized that I had it backward my entire life! No blame or shame. I learned this to survive. I had to create certainty and safety around me. I had to do that as a child. And those beliefs persisted far beyond the time I truly needed those strategies to cope with my reality. Forcing my life into a specific shape that I perceived would create the conditions for my happiness never worked, or it never worked well enough anyway!

So, while it seemed initially that learning about his imminent death was a terrible reality that Harold Crick needed to face, it turned out that everything was working out for him as he began to live differently from a place of simply wanting to feel good. He traveled so far in his mindset from the beginning of the movie to the end. This is the moment-to-moment journey of your life. Allow yourself to respect how you are feeling and how far you've come. It takes courage to consider the possibility of making a big leap into what seems like an abyss of uncertainty. Know that there is so much waiting for you on the other side!

What Happens When You Have the Courage to Take the Leap

- You will understand that you are worthy to make decisions to do what you want to do.
- You will feel full emotional freedom in your life.
- You will have more energy and mental clarity as you create more coherent signaling in your body and mind.
- You will recover from your illnesses and symptoms.
- You will choose vitality and joy in your life, and fully understand that vitality is a choice.
- You will create work that doesn't feel like work.
- You will work in your zone of creative genius bringing to the forefront your unique gifts and talents.
- If you have children, you will model for your children how to make decisions in integrity with your needs.

- You will have the tools to provide healing to others in a genuinely holistic way from a space of fullness and true love rather than overwhelming depletion.
- You will feel great!

Daydream about what your dream life looks like. Start there if you can. When you begin to believe it is possible, then you can start to step into the beauty and excitement of uncertainty to free yourself from a life of seemingly endless obligations, to create a life that feels good and satisfying to you. This is your purpose: to awaken and to be happy and content.

Chapter 11:

Sounds Great, but You're Still Not Sure You Can Quit Your Job

*"Without leaps of imagination or dreaming we
lose the excitement of possibilities.
Dreaming, after all is a form of planning."*
– Gloria Steinem

A Story of Taking the Leap

Sarah Knight is a freelance writer who gave an amazingly well-delivered TEDx talk in 2017 on "The Magic of Not Giving a F***," which has, to date, over six million views. If you haven't watched it, watch it because it's a fun and light-hearted look at how we force ourselves unnecessarily to do the things we don't want to do. This is an excerpt from her talk in which she describes deciding to leave her job:

Two and a half years ago, I was a senior editor at a major New York publishing house. I had spent fifteen years clawing my way up the corporate ladder, I had a roster of best-selling authors, and everything I always thought I wanted from my career was coming to pass. But I was really, really unhappy. The kind of unhappy that makes it hard to get out of bed in the morning; the kind of unhappy that makes it hard to commute forty-five minutes on the New York City subway and hard to spend eight to ten hours at your desk before turning around, going home, and doing it all over again. So, I quit. And making that decision was also really hard. A lot of red wine, a lot of tears. But what came after I quit was nothing short of life-changing. Once I removed myself from the culture and lifestyle of a job that had been making me so unhappy, I was free to focus my time and energy on what would make me happy, including working, but just in a different way, and eventually, moving from Brooklyn to a tropical island.

Sarah Knight now lives in Brooklyn and the Dominican Republic and works happily and freely for herself.

Sounds Great, but You Still Don't Think You Can Do It

I would not be at all surprised if you've read to this point and are still thinking that this all sounds great, and you still don't think you can do it. All of this woo-woo talk about worthiness, self-love, limiting beliefs, and being comfortable with uncertainty is all good and well. However, you may still feel like I don't understand your situation, and how you don't think you can quit your job to create a life that you love. I get it. Remember, I'm the Asian chick who did everything in her power not to quit the job that was killing her more and more quickly.

Know that I am not in any way telling you what to do in your life. Your life is your life, and you have the freedom to do with it whatever you want. Whoa. Did you hear what I said? *Your life is your life, and you have the freedom to do with it whatever you want.* That means, of course, that you can choose to stay where you are doing what you are doing. It's no one else's business if you decide to stay where you are.

Yet, the key to creating the life that you want is first to turn down the volume on the things that keep you in a chronic state of survival and then decluttering your mind. Ultimately, when you ask yourself the right questions about where you are and the problems you are facing, you will find yourself slowly, and sometimes quickly, moving to live a happy and satisfying life as you are meant to live, as we all are meant to live. All of this talk about worthiness, self-love, limiting beliefs, etc. is to help you to eventually get to a place where you can make decisions from your heart, honoring your deepest needs. Then, your inner life and outer life will match each other. It requires that you know what you need and want, and then move toward creating a life that matches your needs and desires.

How Do You Want to Spend the Currency of Your Life: Your Time, Energy, and Money?

Further along in her TEDx talk, Sarah Knight talks about the necessity of "mental decluttering" to create space for the life she really wanted to live. She defines currency of our lives as our time, energy, and money, and she very elegantly describes how to take back your time, energy, and money by decluttering your mind by using something she calls "The Not Sorry Method" of being honest and polite about what you do and don't want to do in your life. Ultimately, what she is talking about is being truly authentic in your life and not promising to do things just because you want to please or not disappoint others in your life. However, after you watch the talk, you might have objections arise in your head like I did when I watched it (even now, I can still see some of my old mental programming come up!):

- You probably don't have kids.
- You probably have more support around you than I do.
- You probably don't have a significant history of trauma that completely distorts your sense of worthiness and self-love.
- You probably don't have a history of anxiety and depression.
- You probably have a financial cushion that allowed you to make that decision to quit your job and move to a tropical island.
- You don't have the problems that I have in my life.

While it is entirely valid to have all of the feelings that you have about how hard it would be to decide to quit your job, *know that the cost of not leaving is even higher*. So, even though I can still observe some of my conditioned habits of mind come up from time to time, the point is that I watch my thoughts now. Because I can watch my thoughts, I now know that *I am not my thoughts!* The pause between feelings, thoughts, and actions gives me the freedom to make choices from a well-considered place instead of merely acting from a place of fearful reactivity. I ultimately had a reckoning with myself to consider my worthiness, sense of self-love, my limiting beliefs, and my massive discomfort with uncertainty. And I leaped and left my job. It was the best decision for me.

You Don't Believe You're Brave Enough

Many, many people have told me that I was brave to leave my job as an OB/GYN. Sure I was! Did I know what was ahead? Not really. I had the plan to build my functional medicine practice, and I did. And that was a pretty hefty goal given that I had never owned a business and that I was planning to practice medicine and offer care in an entirely new way. Having a definite plan was not what made it possible for me to leave my job. As Gloria Steinem said, it was the dreaming that was the planning. It was knowing that the cost of not leaving my job had become too high. What is the cost to you of not leaving your job? And how far will you let it go before you literally can't work anymore?

What Is Your Precious Life Worth to You?

Your life is immeasurably valuable to you and those around you. You are first in line for yourself. We talked about why putting on your oxygen mask is so vitally important. It's not merely that when you take care of yourself that you are then better able to take care of others. Of course, this is part of the picture. The most important reason is that life can only really feel good when you are living in complete integrity with yourself. When you continually consider the needs of others as more important than your own, you will invariably experience ongoing negative emotions that don't feel good at all. The constant negative emotions provide the information you need to know that you are not acting for yourself. When you continually act against yourself from a stance of chronic fear and survival, you will have incoherent signaling within your body, and you will get more sick and tired. And you may be thoroughly sick and tired of being sick and tired just as I was.

So, what do you say?

Start by Being Curious

If the only thing that changes after reading this book is that you begin to be curious and start to notice your feelings, thoughts, and emotions without judgment (not easy, I know), then that's a good start.

If you feel as if you are ready to move forward with feeling better and then maybe even choosing work that feels good and in complete alignment with your needs and wants, then this is a great place to start!

Start Walking toward What You Want, and You Will Be Helped Along the Way

What can you expect when you start to take steps to move in the direction of feeling better? You will notice that seemingly "accidental" things will begin to happen to support you. This is because when you start to change the way you think about things, the things around you start to change, as the spiritual teacher Wayne Dyer taught over and over again. "If you change the way you look at things, the things you look at will change." He said it over and over again because it's true, and he wanted everyone to know that this is the truth, the way things are.

When Bill Moyers interviewed the famous American mythologist Joseph Campbell in 1988, he asked him: *"Do you ever have the sense of... being helped by hidden hands?"* And Joseph Campbell answered:

All the time. It is miraculous. I even have a superstition that has grown on me as a result of invisible hands coming all the time – namely, that if you do follow your bliss, you put yourself on a kind of track that has been there all the while, waiting for you, and the life that you ought to be living is the one you are living. When you can see that, you begin to meet people who are in your field of bliss, and they open doors to you. I say, follow your bliss and don't be afraid, and doors will open where you didn't know they were going to be.

If you continue to live the life you are living from a place of fear and survival, then you will never give yourself the opportunity to meet other people who can help you on your path. You can only live what you know. So, start moving in the direction of what you don't know! When you begin to live your life on purpose from a place of complete authenticity, from the position of not caring about the things that don't matter to you, the beauty of your life will start to unfold. You will feel better than you ever imagined possible. You'll believe it when you see it. And then you will continue to see it when you continue to believe it. Follow your bliss!

Chapter 12:

You've Got This! If I Can Do It, You Can Too!

*"Our deepest fear is not that we are inadequate.
Our deepest fear is that we are powerful
beyond measure.
It is our light, not our darkness that most
frightens us.
We ask ourselves, 'Who am I to be brilliant,
gorgeous, talented, fabulous?'
Actually, who are you not to be?
You are a child of God.
You playing small does not serve the world.
There is nothing enlightened about shrinking
so that other people won't feel insecure*

around you.
We are all meant to shine, as children do.
We were born to make manifest the glory of God
that is within us.
It's not just in some of us; it's in everyone.
And as we let our own light shine,
we unconsciously give other people permission
to do the same.
As we are liberated from our own fear,
our presence automatically liberates others."
–Marianne Williamson

Shine, Baby, Shine!

You've likely heard this very famous passage from Marianne Williamson's book, *A Return to Love.* What she is describing so well is a form of the "upper limit problem" we discussed in Chapter 9 about limiting beliefs and what holds us back from taking the leap from anything we know well to something we don't. What lies underneath this problem is that we often stick desperately to what we know because we believe that this is what keeps us safe and alive. It's a limited tolerance for feeling good that is born from deep fears about what will happen if we dare to move beyond the well-cultivated and planned paths that we are on now. Know that when you begin to step toward the life you want to live, you will start to shine more brightly and find the energy and clarity to live the life you ought to be living.

Your Fear Is Real, and You Can Liberate Yourself From that Fear

One of the first things that I wanted to validate for you in this book is that the fear you are feeling about making new and unfamiliar choices is real. The multiple causes and conditions that have led to your life as one overflowing with responsibilities, exhaustion and over-whelm originated from your own need for a sense of pre-dictability and safety in your life. It seemed that the best way to do that was to become a doctor with a noble and good intention to help others. What you may not have known was that the ongoing need for predictability and safety is what has been creating the endless cycles of feeling worse despite your many attempts to feel better. Moreover, the container of the practice of medicine also does not provide the conditions for you to feel safe or calm; instead, the ongoing and increasing pressures of medical practice contribute to your feelings of unwell-ness and getting sick.

At the start of the book, we took a disturbing look into how many doctors are feeling about the stress and over-whelm of practicing medicine, and how nearly half of all doctors surveyed were planning to change career paths. I also talked about the alarmingly higher rate of suicide among doctors and especially among female physicians. I could have been one of those who successfully took her own life. You picked up this book because you haven't been feeling well. You may be feeling burned out and exhausted. You are one of the many doctors who have considered leaving your job because you are so unhappy, sick, and oh so, so tired.

I shared with you my own story of recurring crazy and stress, and it wasn't easy to write about any of that. It took me back to the many feelings I had during that time of feeling trapped, powerless, unseen, and sad. Yet, I wrote through feeling all of those feelings for one reason: to let you know that you are not alone. It is okay and safe to talk about not feeling good and how crazy it has been for you walking this tightrope and living this life of being every woman to everyone.

Do you think I ever had any intention or goal to tell anyone about the darkest times of my life while I was practicing conventional medicine, to admit how sick I had become during that time? Not at first. And when I began to first claw my way out of the hole that had become my life back into the light, I realized that I had no reason to feel the unrelenting shame that I felt for so long. When I was able to accept the parts of myself that were trying to save me, I was ready to start to have some compassion for the suffering person who just wanted the severe pain to end, the pain of living a life completely out of alignment with my own needs and wants. And yet, I continued to act against myself repeatedly because I did not understand that if I actually could tune into what I needed and listen, then I might be able to feel better. I wanted to tell my story so that you might have the courage to tell your story. Then you can get on the road to feeling better too.

Start with Two Questions

Addressing the real roots of why I was making the decisions I was making and uncovering the core beliefs that I had developed when growing up helped me to ask and contemplate the right questions to return to my fundamental worthiness and self-love. This is not where I started, though. Because my beliefs were centered around the core belief that the needs of others were more important than mine, I began with these questions, and asked you to do the same:

1. Am I doing what I originally intended in my work as a doctor?
2. Am I helping my patients in the ways I know that they need help?

During my process of considering these questions, I pursued further training in integrative medicine and functional medicine. I began to understand more clearly how ongoing chronic stress creates cycles of ongoing incoherent body signaling and then eventually, the symptoms of illness. You learned that sending your body signals of safety and calm by turning down the volume of stress in your body and your surrounding life is foundational to returning to the coherent and aligned functioning in your body. When your body remembers its original state of alignment, you begin to feel better, to have more energy, and to be able to think clearly about your own life.

In Chapter 6, I outlined for you a basic functional medicine approach to address the fundamentals of the imbalance in different body systems. By telling your story and examining the lab data, the physiologic signature of ongoing stress in your body, you will then have the powerful tools and leverage you need to shift your body and mind back to feeling so much better. You will create what you need for ongoing optimal health and wellness. This is where my journey initially began in 2007 after implementing foundational healing practices in my life. By addressing and rebalancing the fundamentals of digestion, detoxification, and neurohormonal signaling, we access the critical leverage we need to relieve most symptoms of illness.

In Chapter 7, you were able to consider what prevents you from choosing to take the best care of yourself. We discussed the first steps to remembering our intrinsic worthiness and self-love, especially for those of us who didn't feel the flow of unconditional love early in our lives.

In Chapter 8, we talked about how we scoff at and ignore the messages to place our oxygen masks on first, how we believe that we can't do that when so many around us depend on us so heavily. Who we believe we are is so intimately intertwined with what we do for others. We become further and further depleted from a distorted sense that if we don't do what we're doing, we won't survive. Yet, acting desperately to fulfill all of the roles will make you sick and affect whatever you thought you were building. You may have been trying to take care of yourself; however, the tools you have been using may hurt you. When you can observe and understand this, you can start to have some genuine caring and compassion for yourself. You can begin to consider what you can do to move out of survival mode, to apply the right and lasting remedies to live your best life.

When you start to care about how you feel and start considering that you might want to quit your job, you will need to look at the limiting beliefs that are holding you back. In Chapter 9, we talked about "upper limit problems." We discussed ways that you can observe and overcome your limiting beliefs to leap to the life you want and deserve, to leave the job that clutters your mind and contributes to ongoing noise of stress and overwhelm.

Taking big leaps in your life requires that you become comfortable with uncertainty, as we discussed in Chapter 10. We examined the idea that becoming comfortable with uncertainty is what creates freedom and a firm and reliable sense of safety. When you can embrace the fact that you are okay in the present moment, right now, and in every subsequent moment, you no longer need external circumstances to meet all of your perceived pre-conditions for happiness, to be able to check off all of the boxes. The truth is that merely checking off all of the boxes does not lead to any lasting happiness because there will always be more boxes to check off. If finding safety is only about checking off boxes and looking for specific outcomes, then there can be no lasting happiness, joy, or satisfaction. When you realize that life is always unfolding for your benefit, even when it initially feels confusing, ugly, and bad, you can start to relax. When you can use all your experiences as your teacher, you will be able to appreciate all aspects of your life. When you can appreciate all aspects of your life, then you can know that you are always okay.

When you can act from a place of knowing that you are okay and feeling good, you will have the power to create the life that you can embrace and love fully. You realize that feeling good comes from within, and you always rely on yourself to feel love and to feel good. This is true freedom. And when you are feeling truly free, you naturally have the energy and mental clarity to live and create precisely what you desire. As you liberate yourself from your fear, your presence liberates others rather than imprisoning them in the trap of your needing things always to look and be a certain way. Your life can unfold in new, exciting, and unexpected ways, and you welcome this because you are now ready to receive whatever comes your way.

In the end, nearly losing my mind and my life were the gifts that allowed me to wake up to my life. Had my life as a conventional OB/GYN been comfortable enough, then I would never have decided to leave and discover true freedom in my life.

My deepest wish for you is to shed who you are now to become who you are meant to be. You have the freedom to choose the life you want. Have the first moment of awareness that you do have the power to make different choices for yourself, as frightening and threatening as making these choices may seem at first. Step by step, you will begin to see and believe what is possible. You will become the author of your life as you want it to be.

To be free and to feel good are what you deserve always.

Acknowledgments

I have been writing books in my mind for quite some time now. As the path and journey of this lifetime unfolded, I never quite had the mental or energetic bandwidth to apply myself to this dream of writing a book until now. I am overflowing with gratitude and appreciation for the opportunity to flow out onto the pages a love letter to all those who have similar experiences.

As I continued to follow my bliss after leaving my conventional medical practice, there were so many teachers and mentors who further opened the doors of consciousness and experience as I could never have imagined before. This is the magic of becoming comfortable with uncertainty and welcoming the excitement of not yet knowing who is going to appear to help you on your path! Infinite blessings and gratitude to my most beloved teachers and mentors.

To my very dear parents, Wendy and Bill Wei, you have been with me through all of it, supporting me with whatever decisions I have made. Thank you for creating and sustaining beauty and growth throughout your lives and mine.

To Ben and David, my Dearest Ones, I am content to know that you are happy and are living amazing lives. Thank you for all you are and are ever becoming. I love you both limitlessly.

Finally, great thanks to Dr. Angela Lauria and the fantastic team at The Author Incubator. Thank you to David Hancock and the Morgan James Publishing team for helping me to create a book that I can share with the world.

Thank You!

Thank you so much for reading *Physician, Care for Thyself: A Doctor's Journey Out of the Darkness of Depression and Burnout.* While it wasn't easy for me to write about some of the darkest moments of my life while practicing as an OB/GYN, I wanted to let you know that you are not alone in the seeming insanity of your struggle.

I would love to know more about your journey, your dreams, and thoughts about leaving your job as a doctor. Please keep in touch! You can reach out to me via email at drwei@jessicaweimd.com.

Let's find your inner Clara Joy, who wants to laugh and play, to be truly free and happy!

About the Author

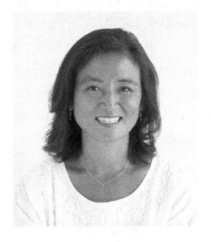

D r. Jessie Wei is a board-certified OB/GYN who had the great privilege and honor to take care of thousands of women for over twenty years. Her conventional medical training began at the University of Virginia School of Medicine, and she completed her residency in Obstetrics and Gynecology at the University of Connecticut School of Medicine.

In search of better questions and keys to healing, she completed her fellowship in Integrative Medicine with the Arizona Center for Integrative Medicine and her certification in Functional Medicine with the Institute for Functional Medicine. After she left her conventional medical practice in 2016, she took the leap to establish her functional medicine practice helping other women find their way back to health, joy, and vitality.

She currently lives in West Hartford, Connecticut with her two sons. She loves to read, write, dance, laugh, prepare, and cook delicious meals, walk barefoot outside, immerse herself in nature, and find freedom in every present moment.

CPSIA information can be obtained
at www.ICGtesting.com
Printed in the USA
JSHW031103241120
9794JS00003B/92